Lo Linkert · Laugh off the pounds

Lo Linkert

LAUGH OFF THE POUNDS

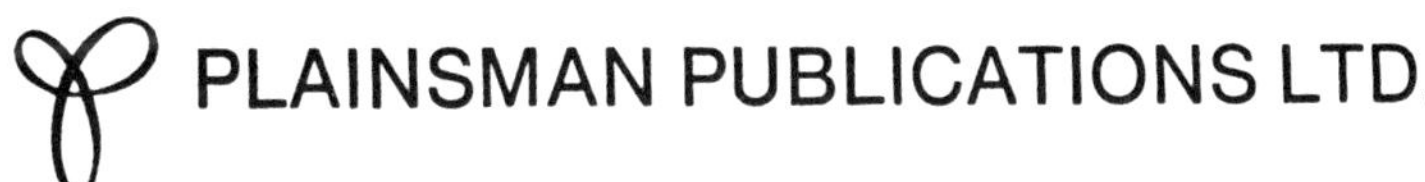
PLAINSMAN PUBLICATIONS LTD.

Published and distributed in Canada by
Plainsman Publications Ltd.
2133 Quebec Street
Vancouver, B.C. V5T 2Z9

Simultaneously published in the U.S. by
Jolex Inc., Oakland, New Jersey and
distributed by John Olson Company
294 West Oakland Avenue
Oakland, New Jersey 07436

Vertrieb für Europa:
Journal-Verlag Schwend GmbH
Schwaebisch Hall, W. Germany

Printed in the U.S.A.
ISBN: 0-89149-059-0

First printing, October 1980

Now that you have purchased this book, congratulations: You have proved that you have a great sense of humor – you are able to laugh at yourself.

Before you go any further, kick off your shoes and relax. Pour yourself a little drink, lean back in your recliner, take a sip, and slowly go from page to page. But don't laugh inside yourself; let it all out! When you finish (if your recliner is still in one piece and you are still able to get up from it), step on the scales. You're on your way to losing weight – with a smile.

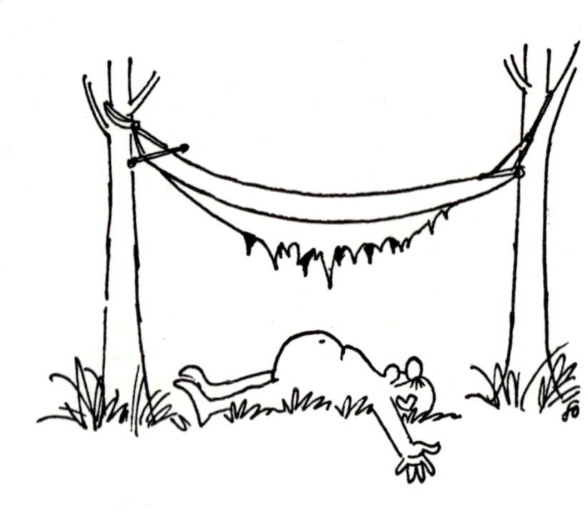

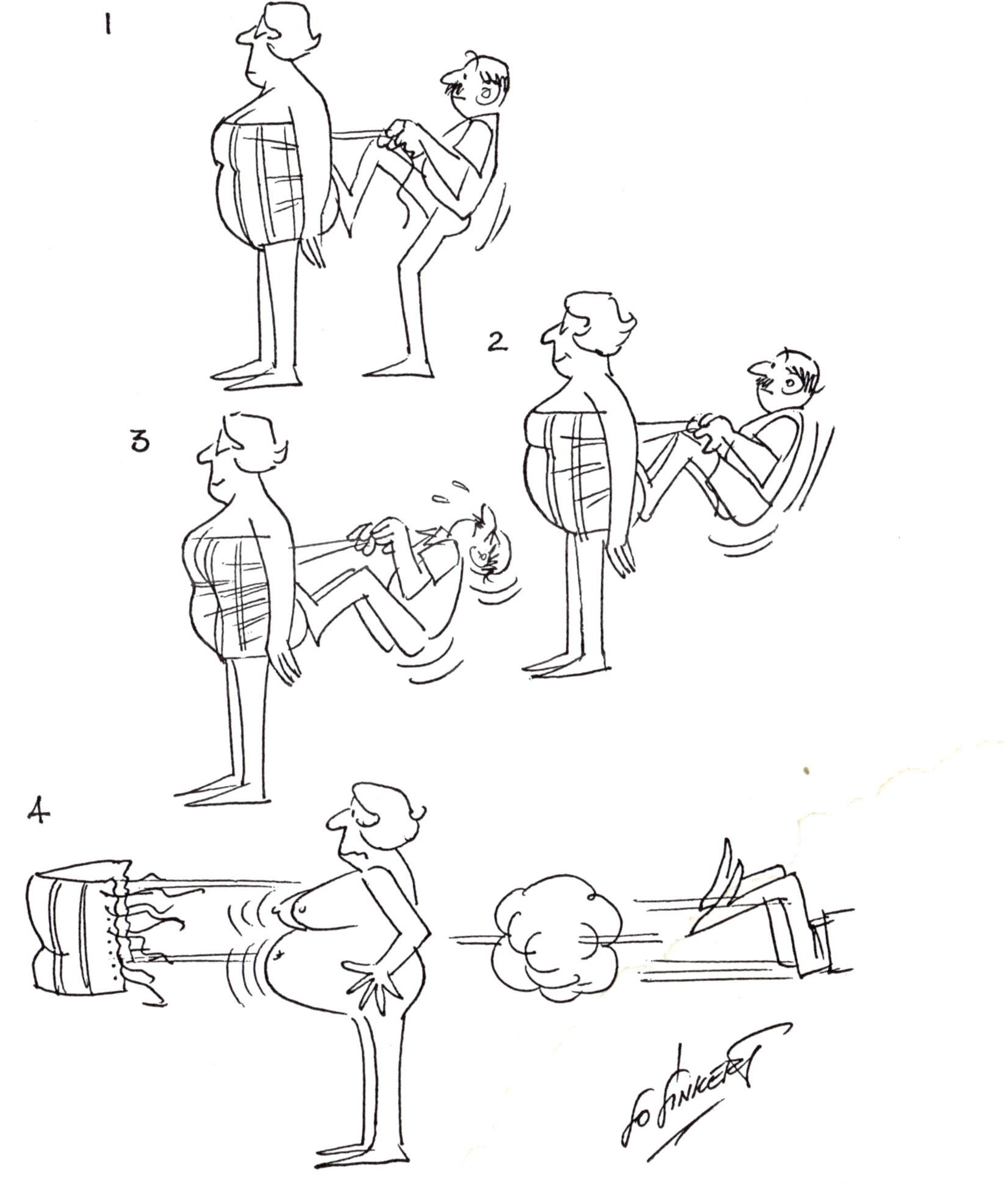
1
2
3
4

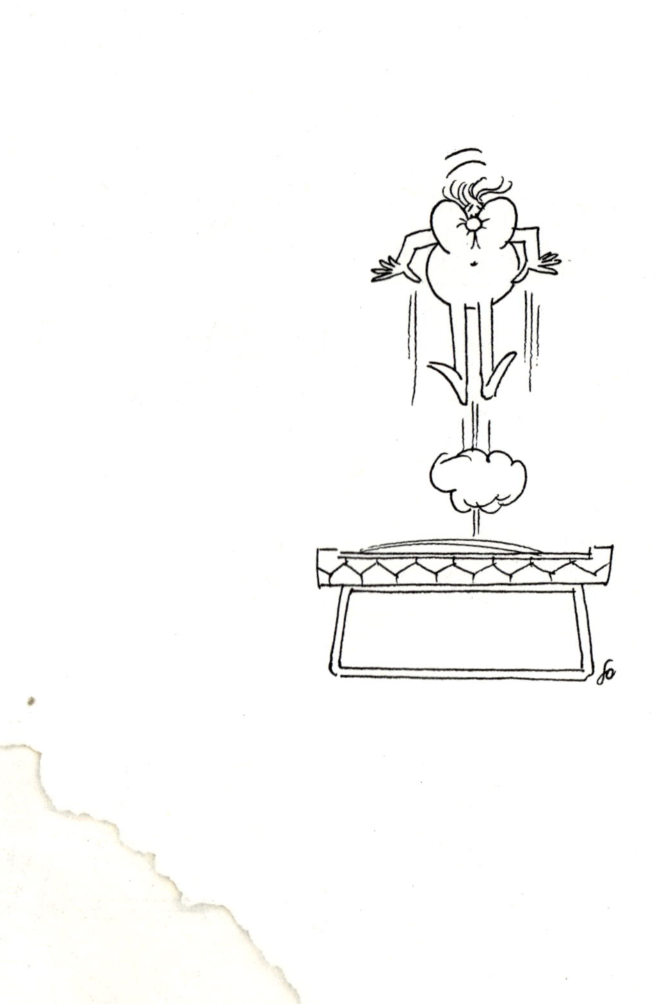

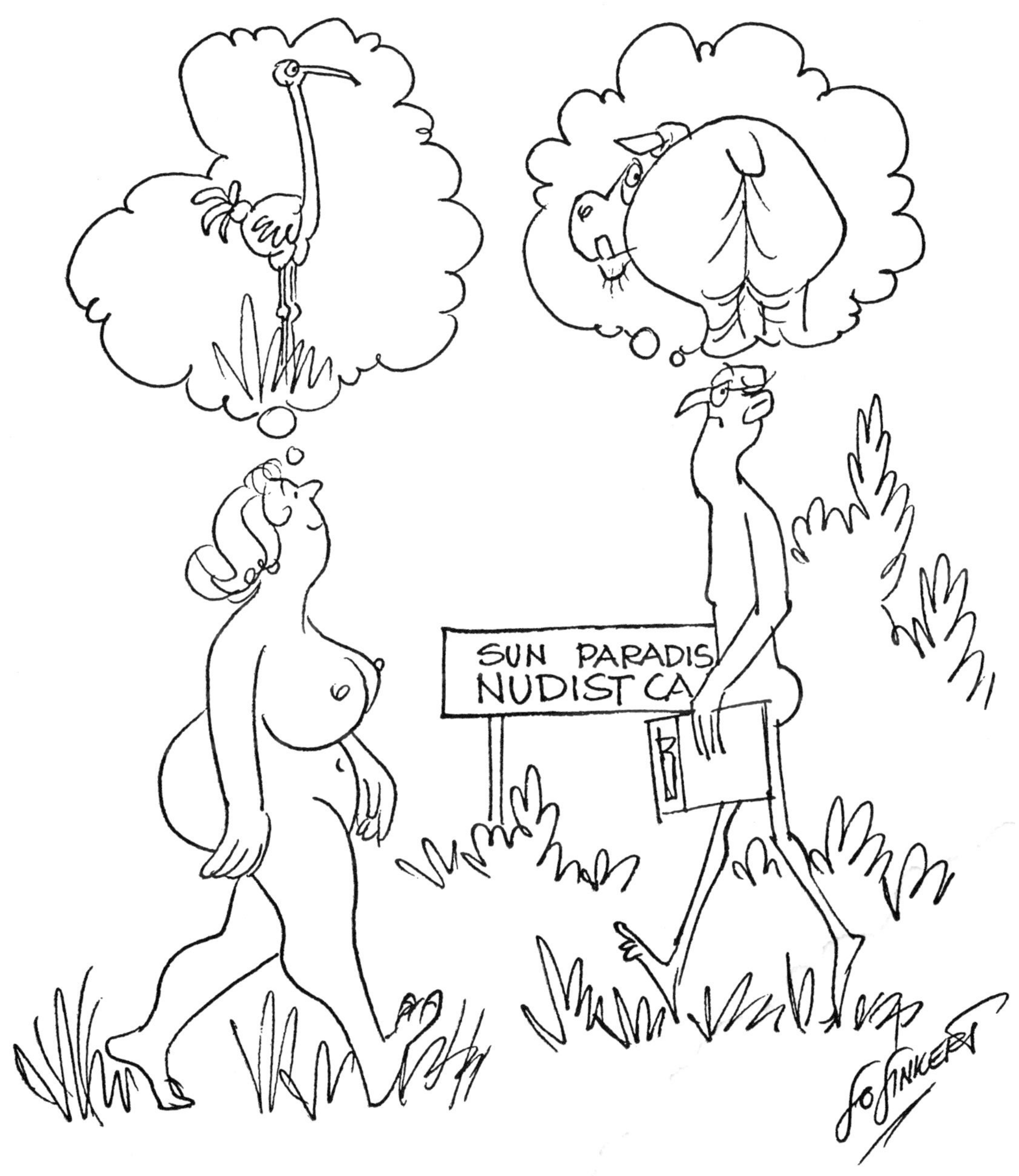
SUN PARADIS
NUDIST CA
JO PINKERT

GOD MADE THE FOOD
BUT THE DEVIL MADE
THE CALORIES.

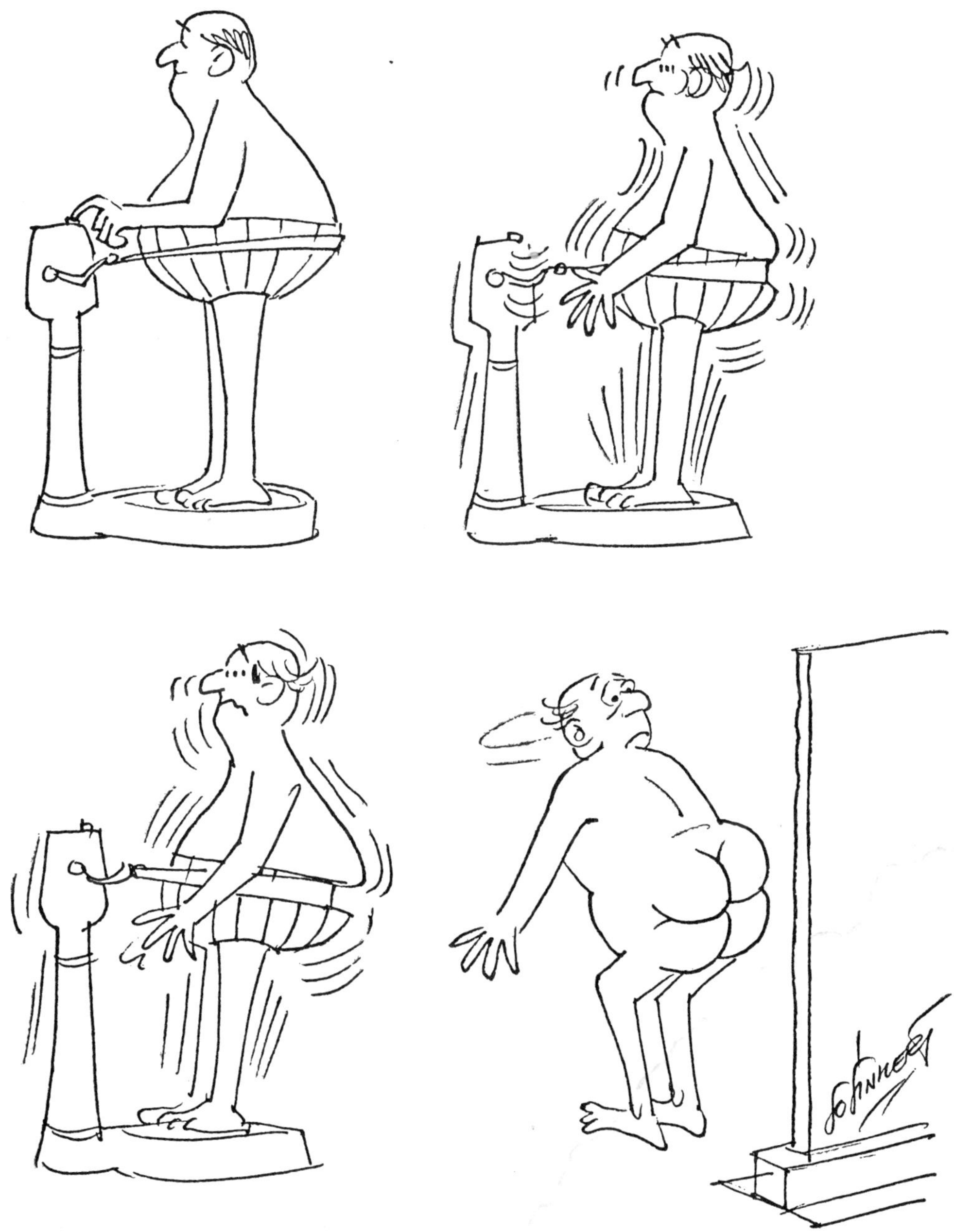

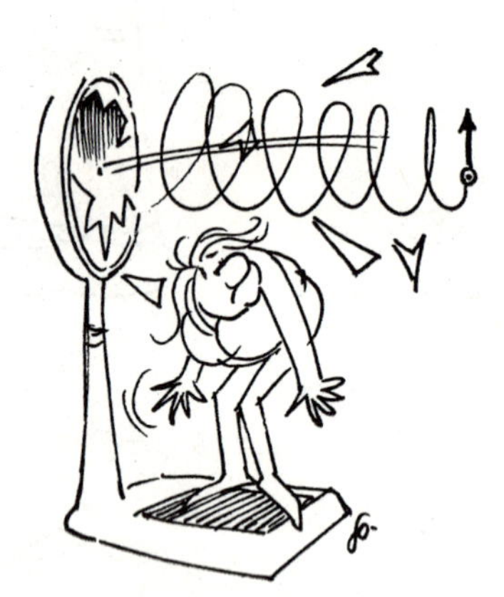

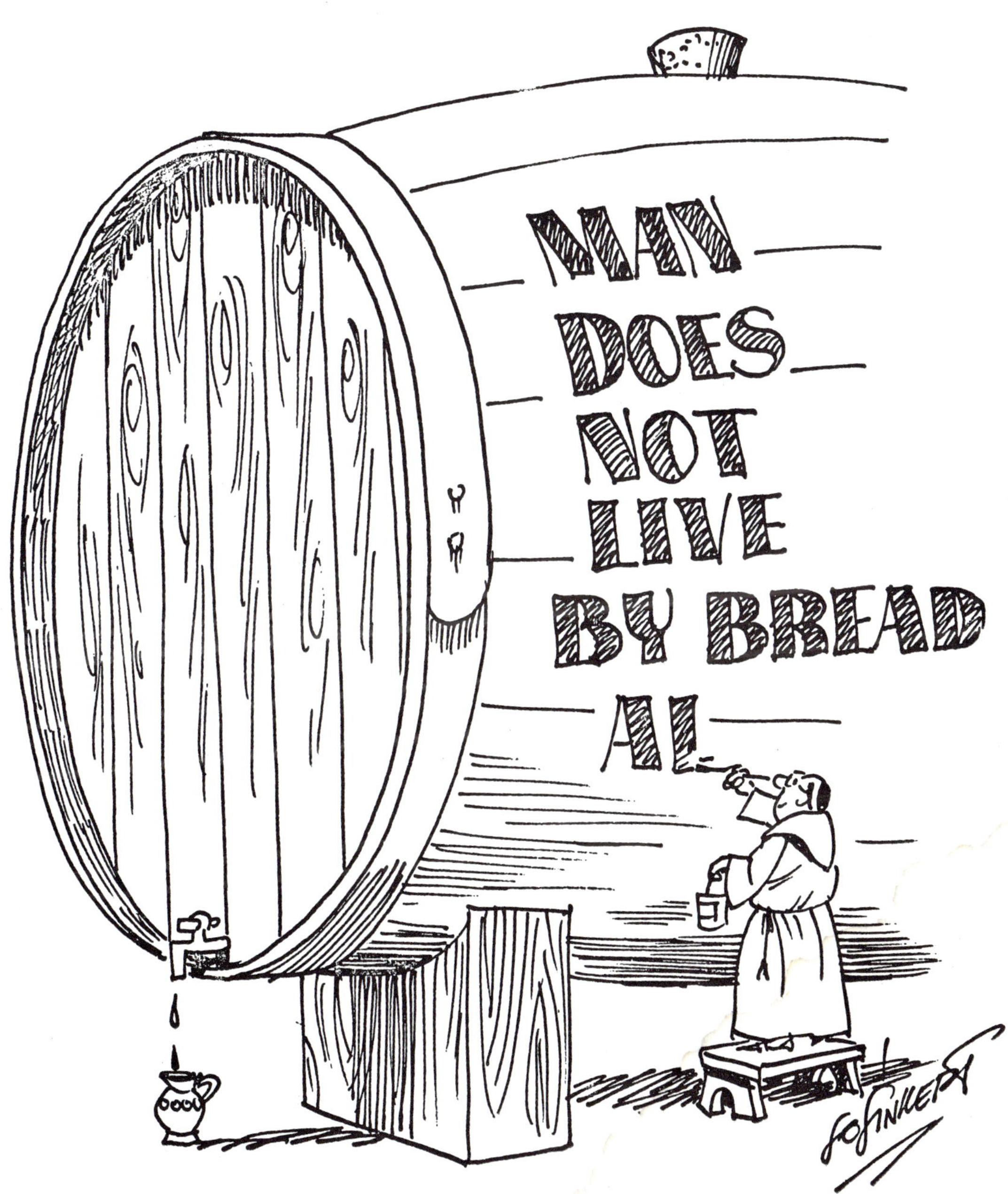
MAN
DOES
NOT
LIVE
BY BREAD
AL

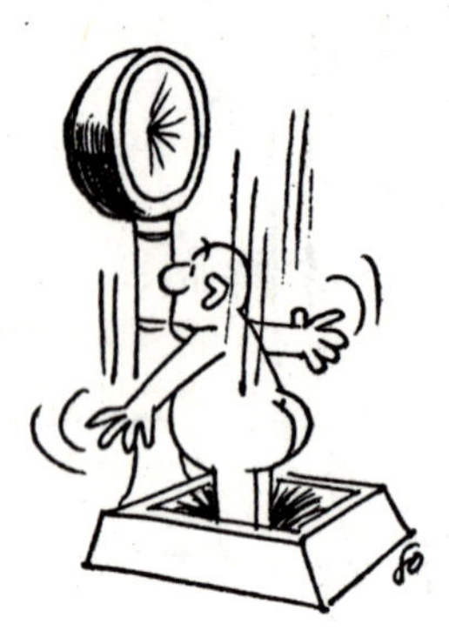

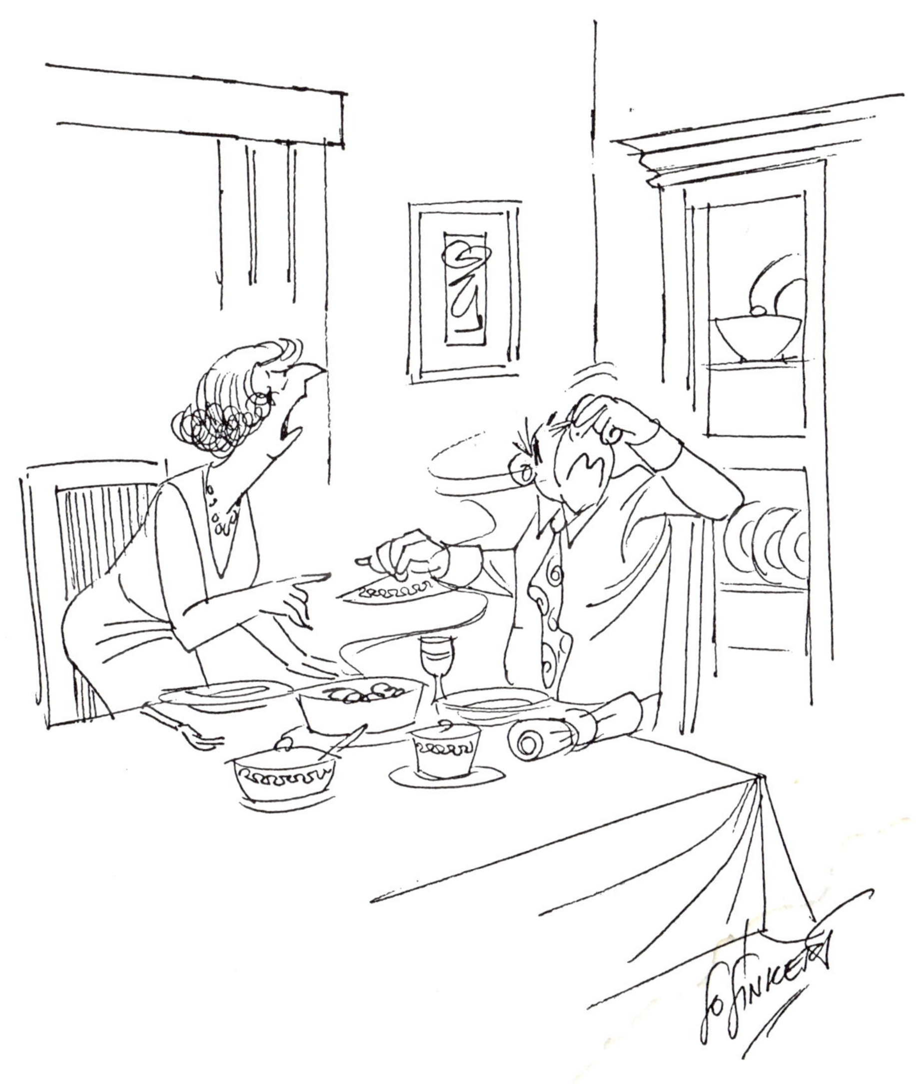

"WHAT'S THE MATTER WITH IT? WHO DO YOU THINK YOU ARE, RALPH NADER?"

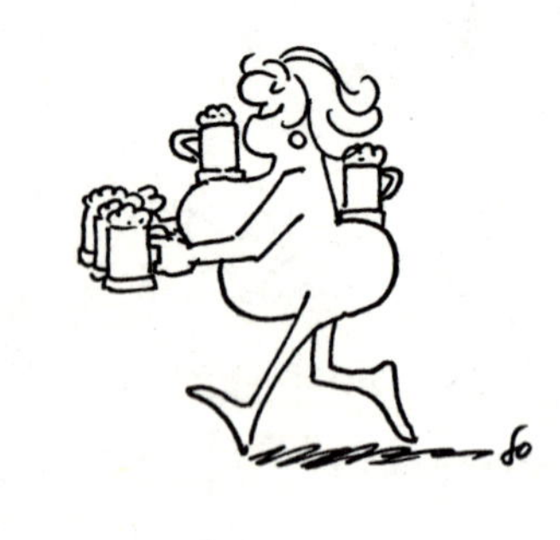

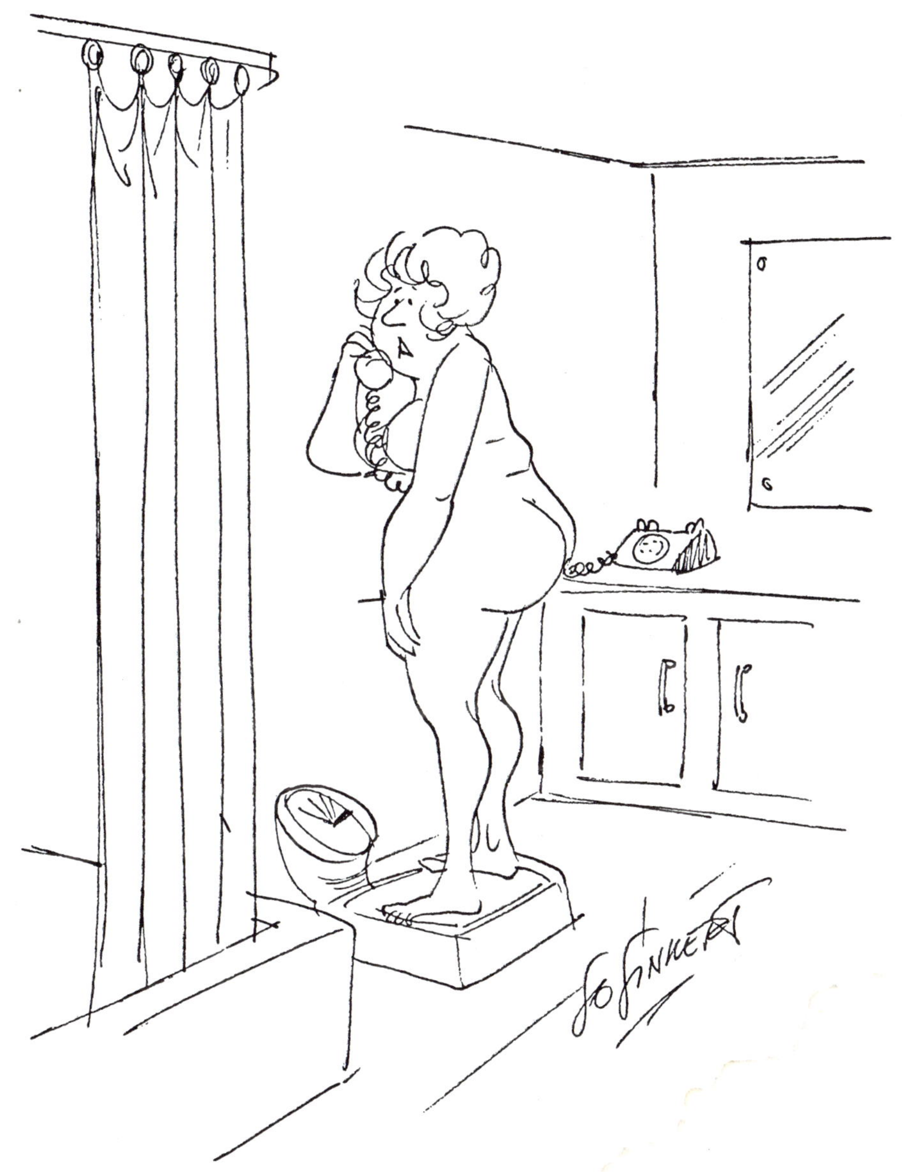

"IS THIS 'DIAL-A-PRAYER'?"

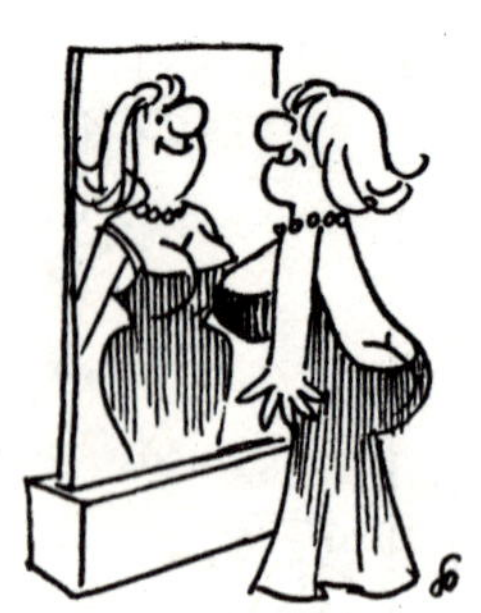

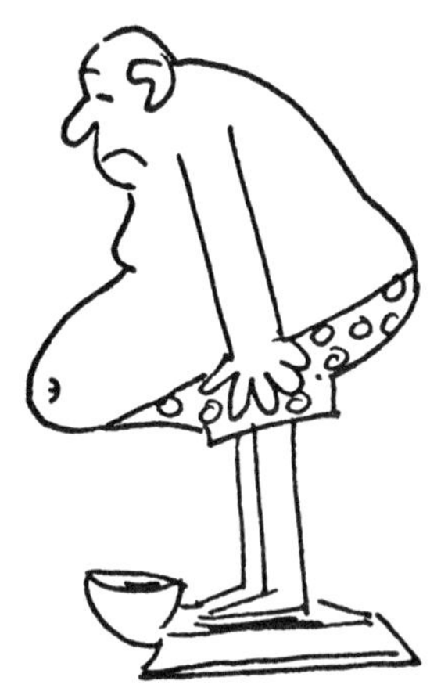

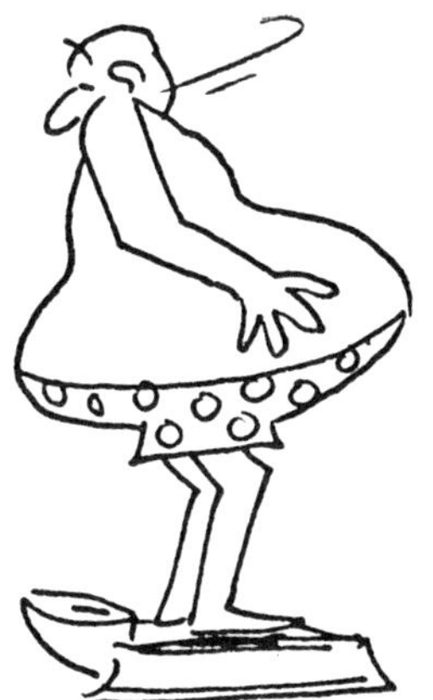

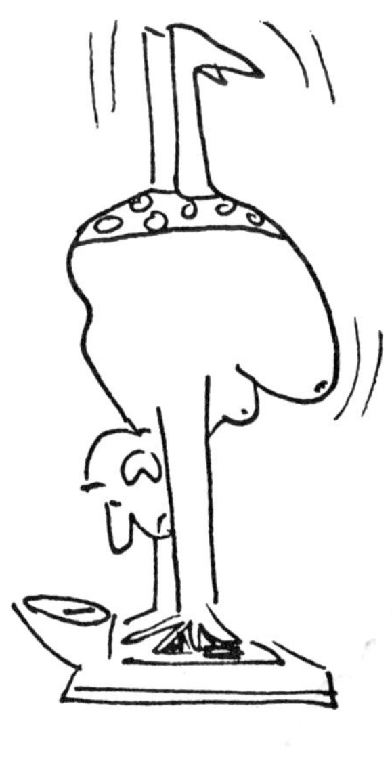

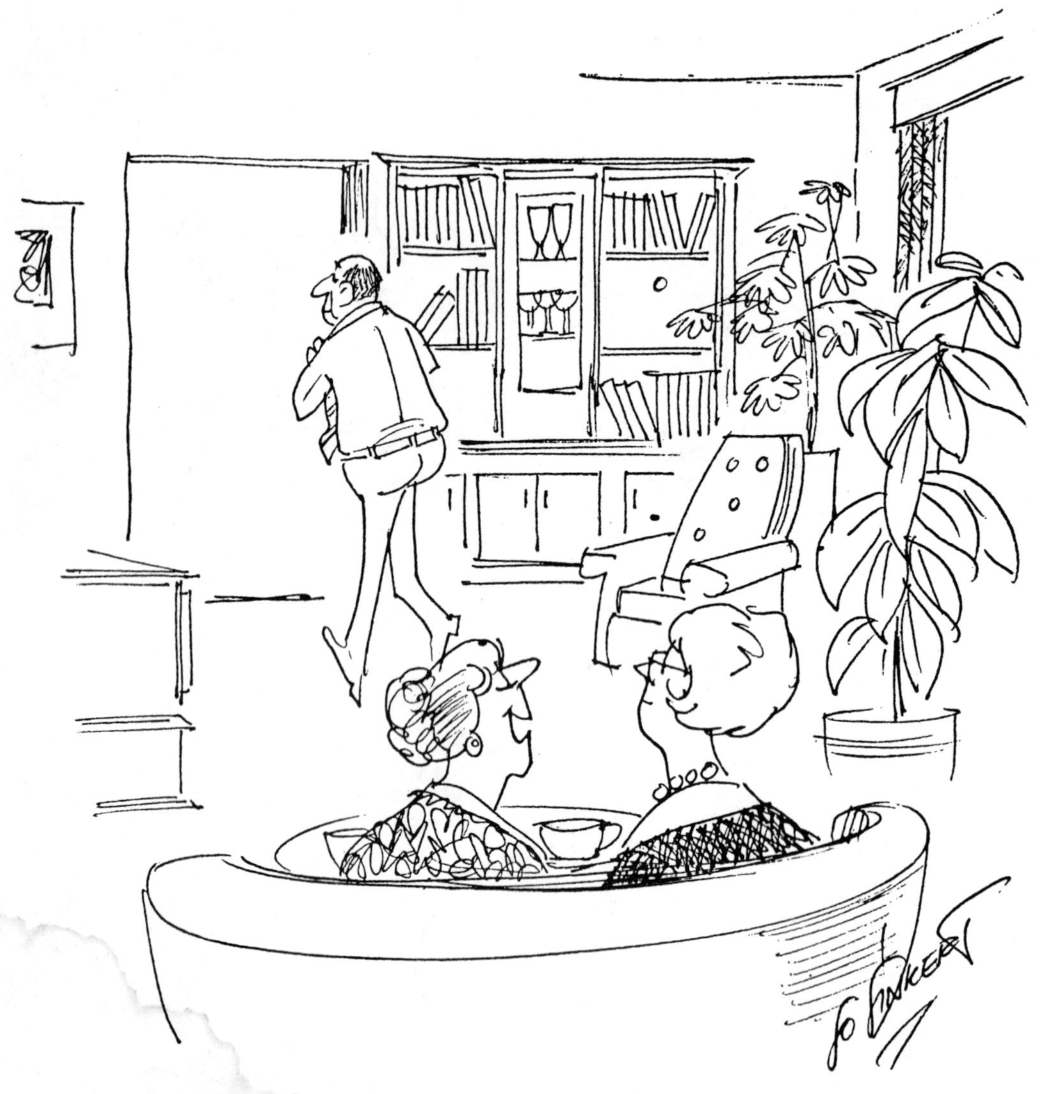

"NOW COMES THE EXCITING PART OF HIS DAY....HE POPS A SHOT OF PRUNE JUICE AND HITS THE SACK."

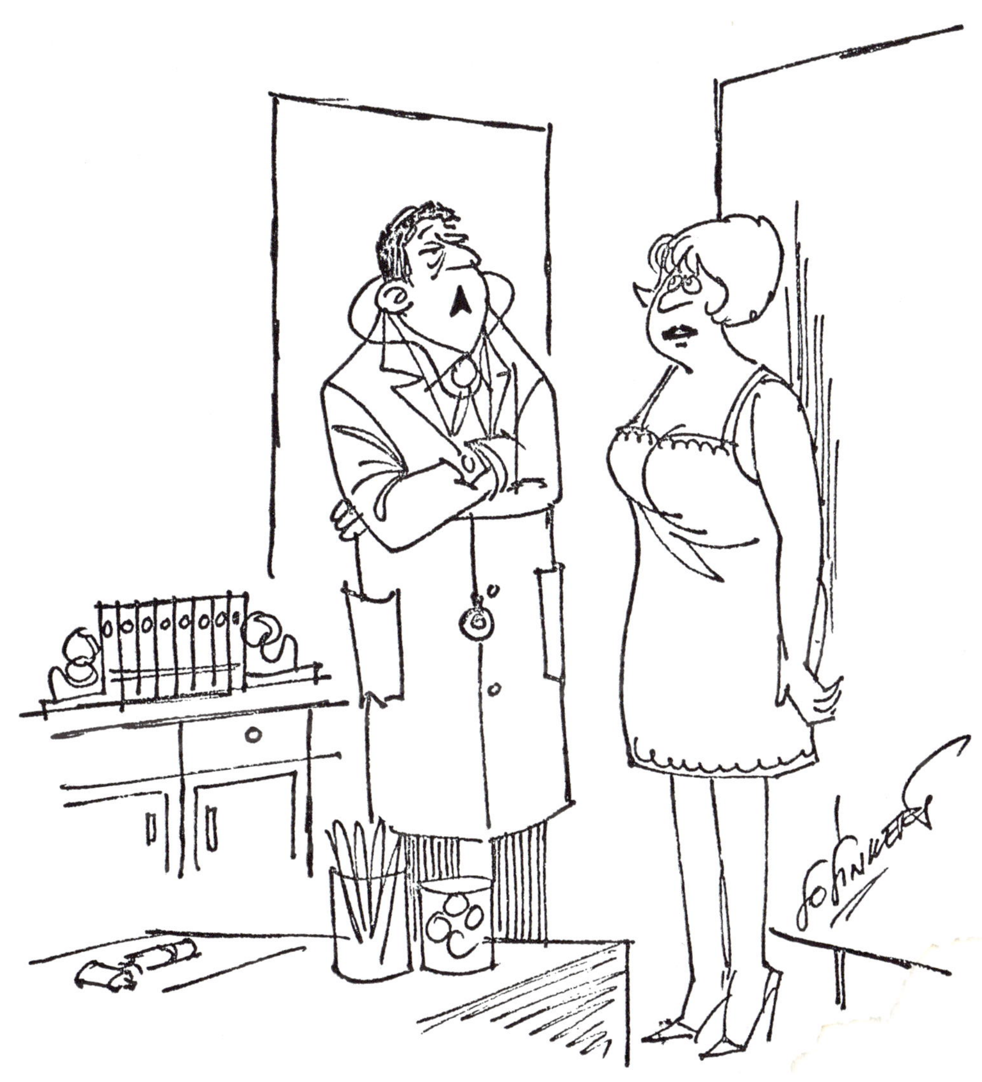

"IF YOU DON'T STOP SPENDING SO MUCH TIME WATCHING THAT 21-INCH SCREEN. YOU'RE GOING TO HAVE A 50-INCH BOTTOM."

IF GOD WANTED US
TO BE SKINNY, HE
WOULDN'T HAVE
GIVEN US STRETCHY
SKIN.

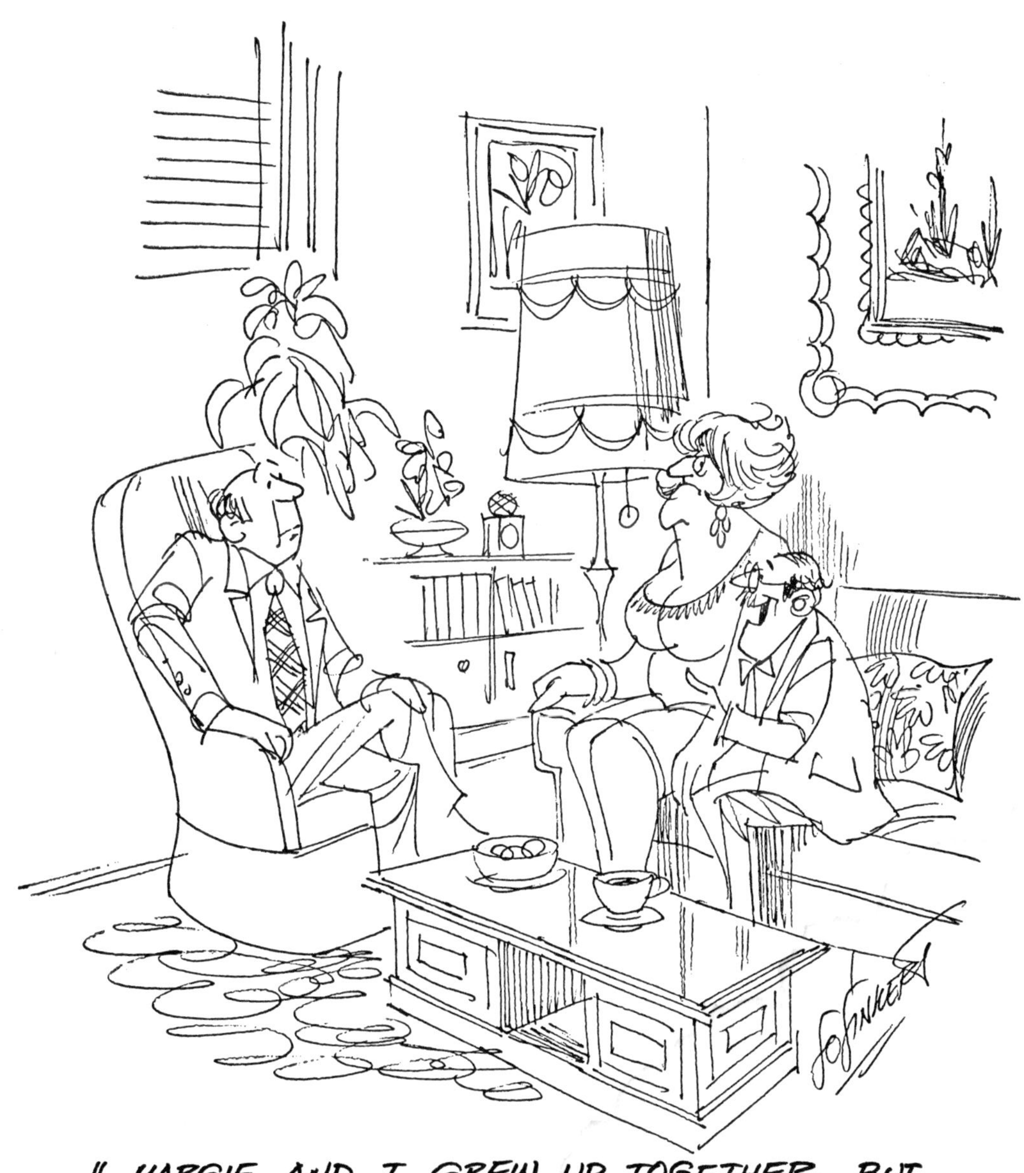

" MARGIE AND I GREW UP TOGETHER, BUT SHE DIDN'T KNOW WHEN TO QUIT. "

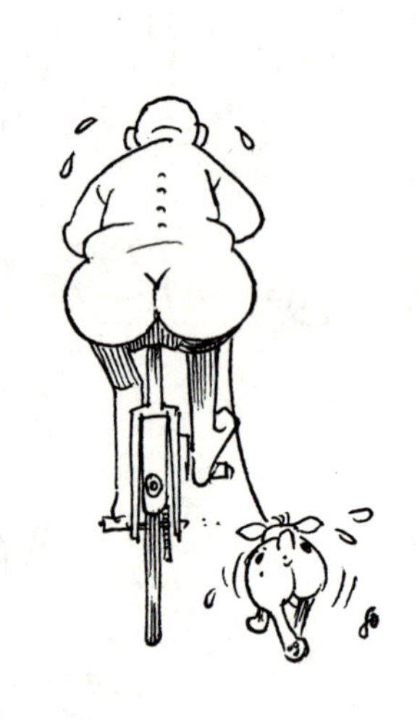

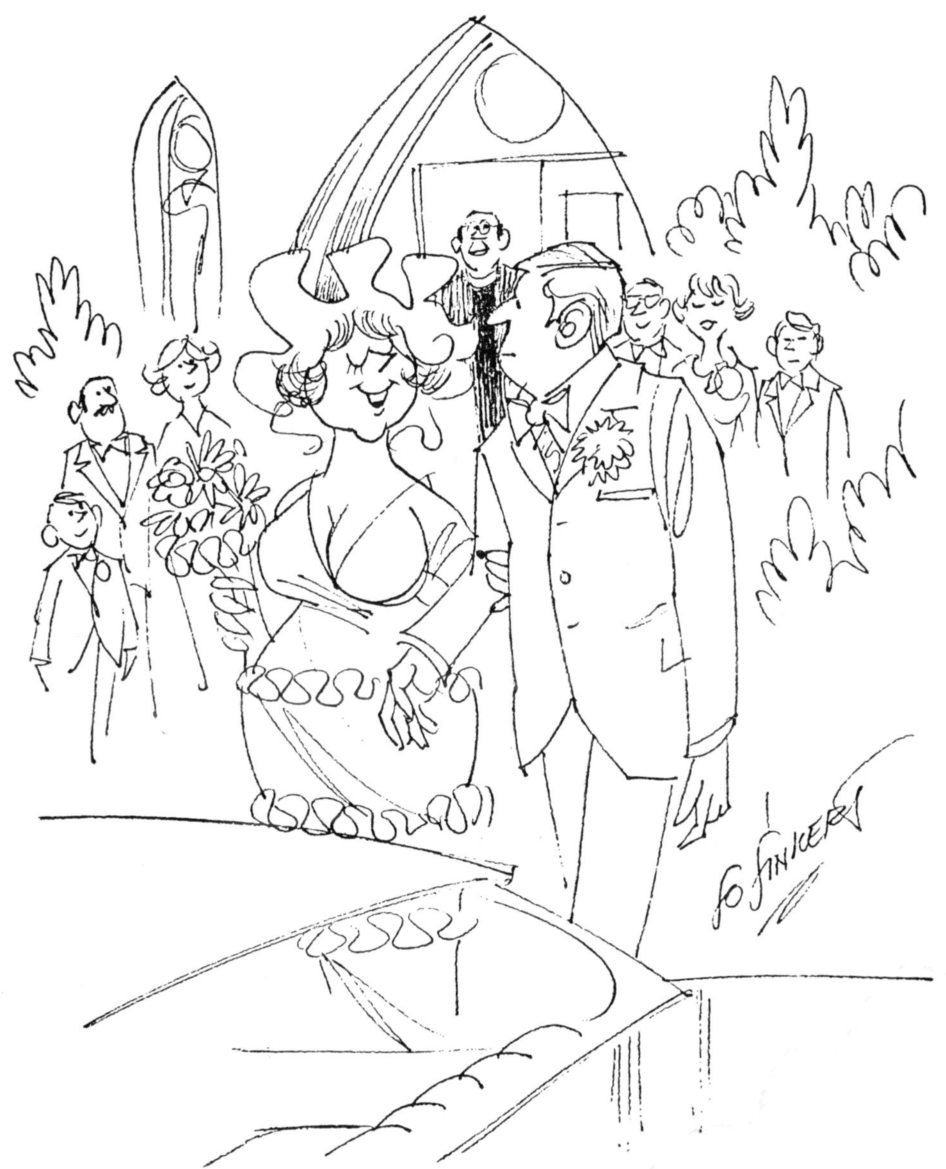

" I CAN'T WAIT UNTIL WE CUT THE CAKE."

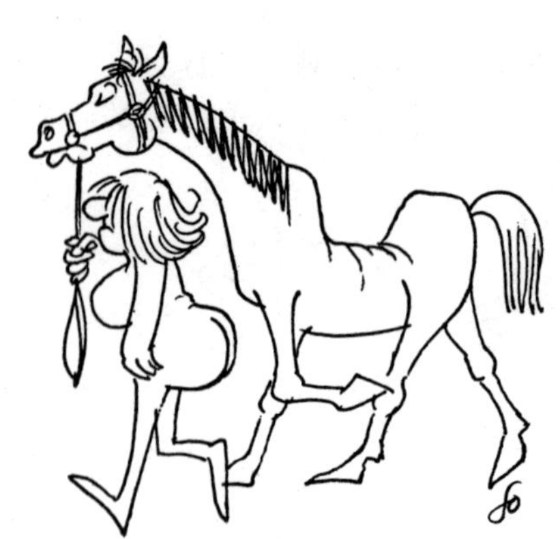

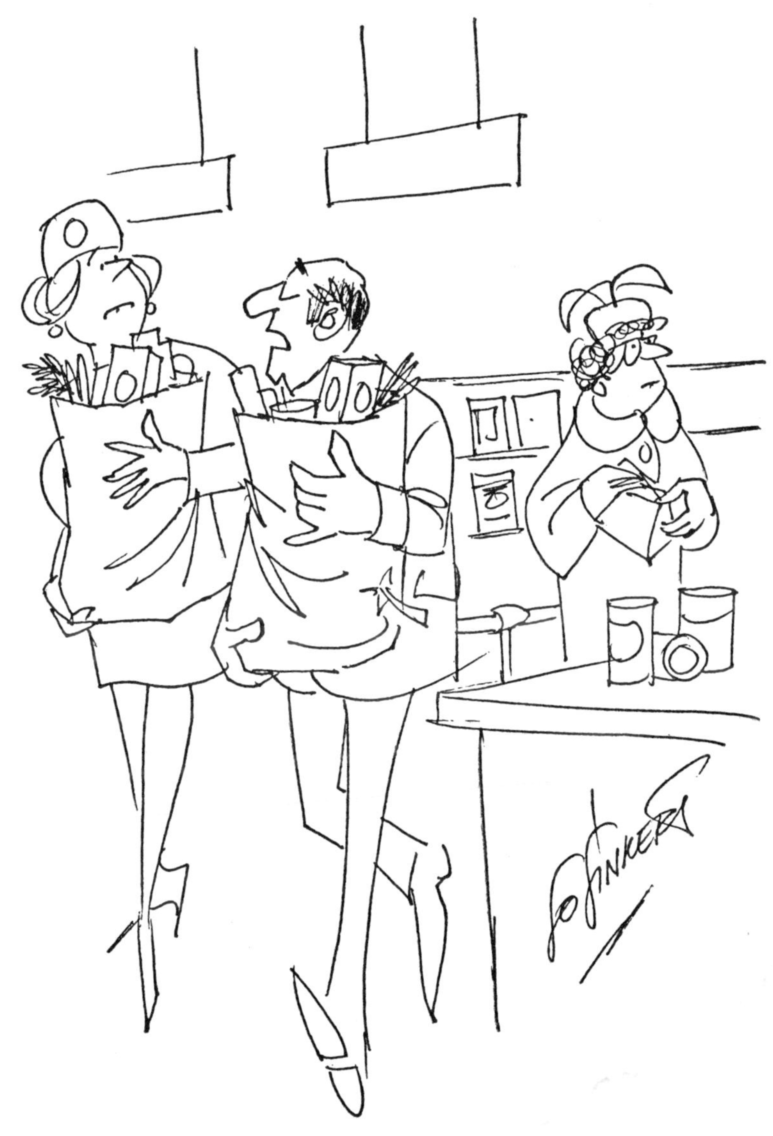

" EITHER WE'RE OVEREATING OR I'M UNDERPAID."

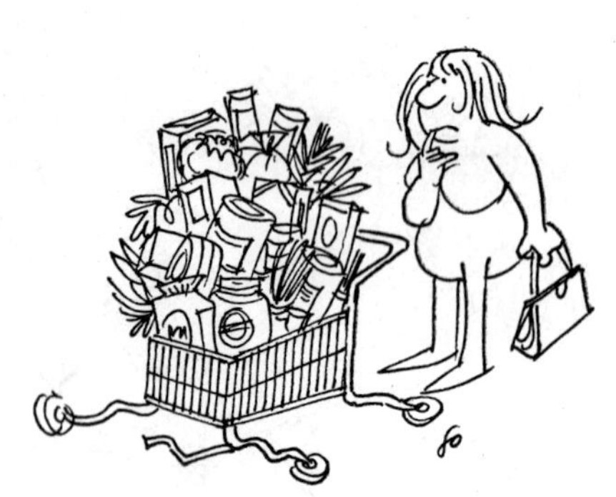

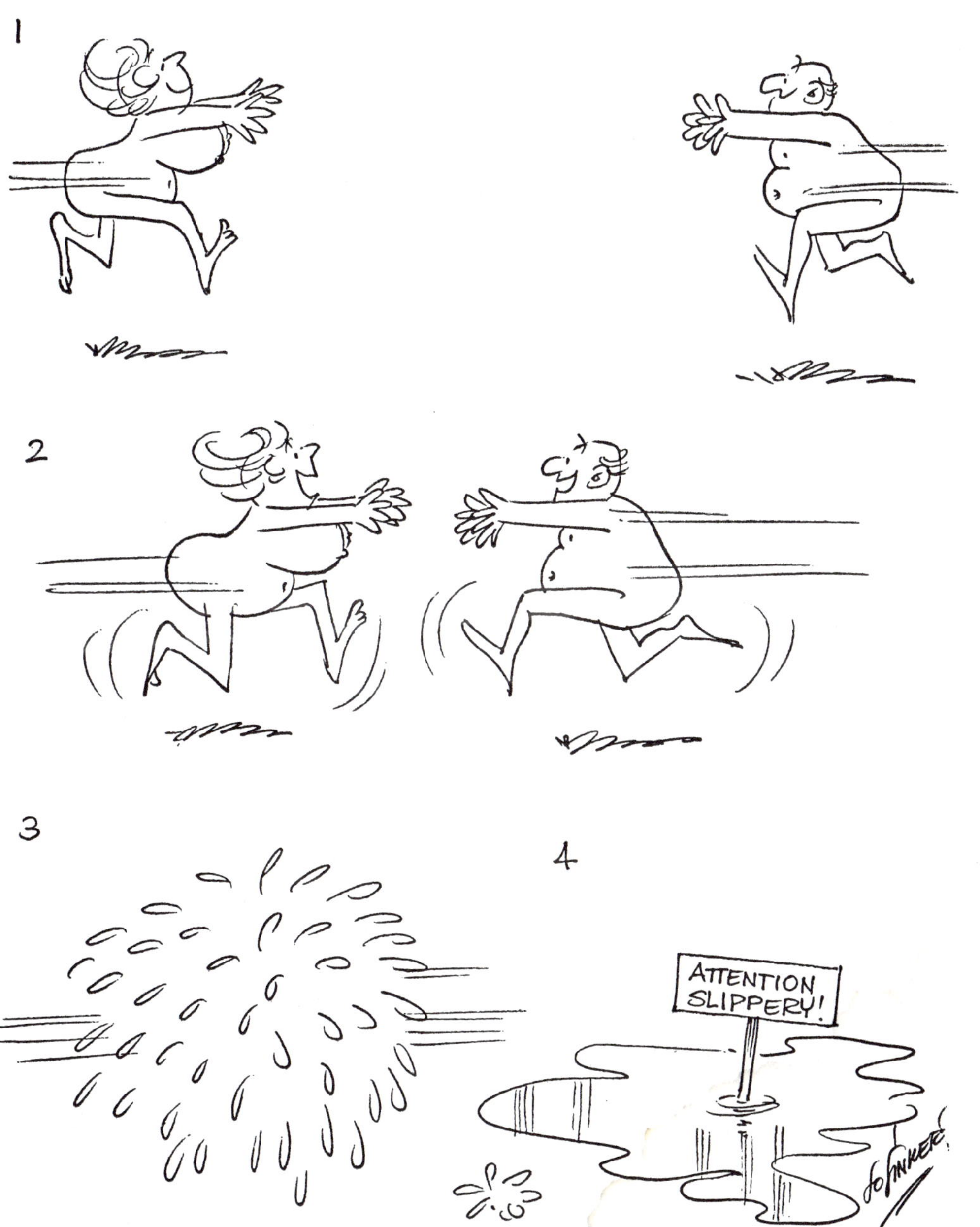
1
2
3
4
ATTENTION
SLIPPERY!

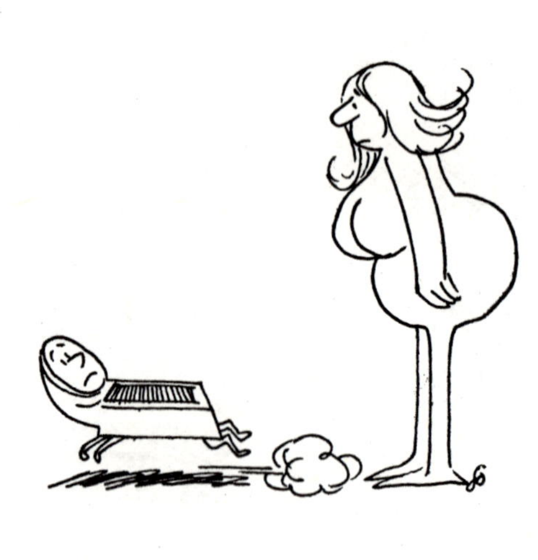

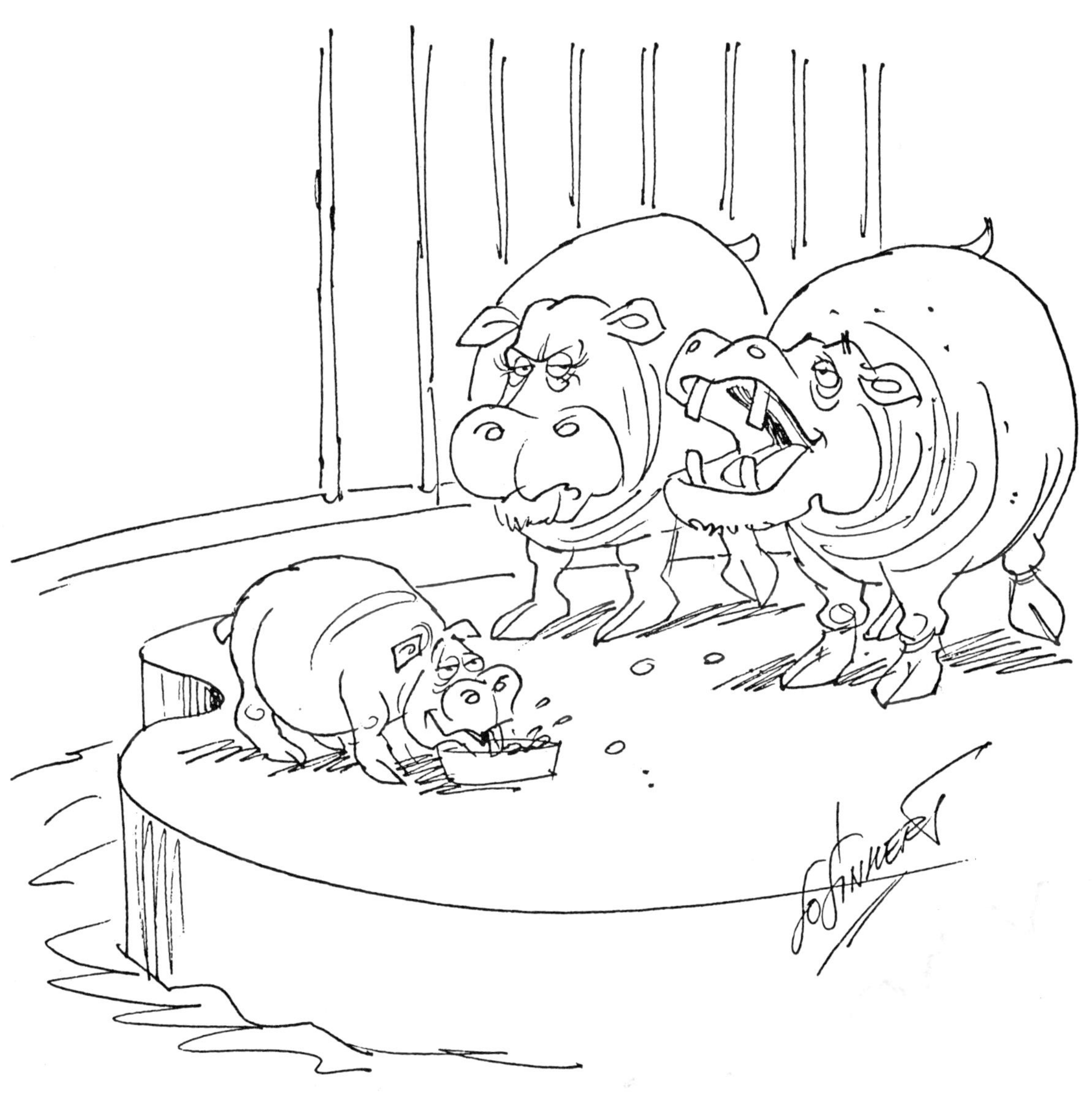

" HE'S GOT MY EYES, AGNES, AND YOUR REAR."

MY PROBLEM IS SPIRALING INFLATION FROM MY BUTT RIGHT UP TO MY DOUBLE CHIN.

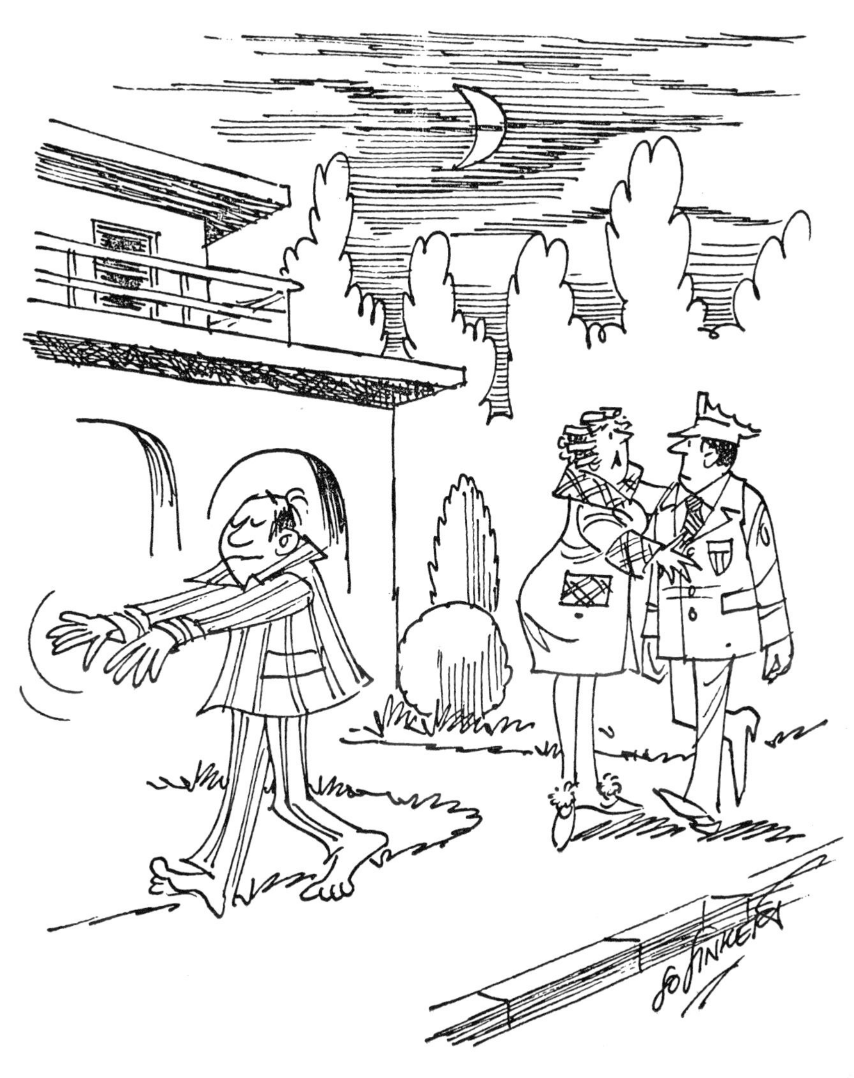

"DON'T DISTURB HIM, OFFICER. HE GETS HIS REST AND EXERCISE AT THE SAME TIME."

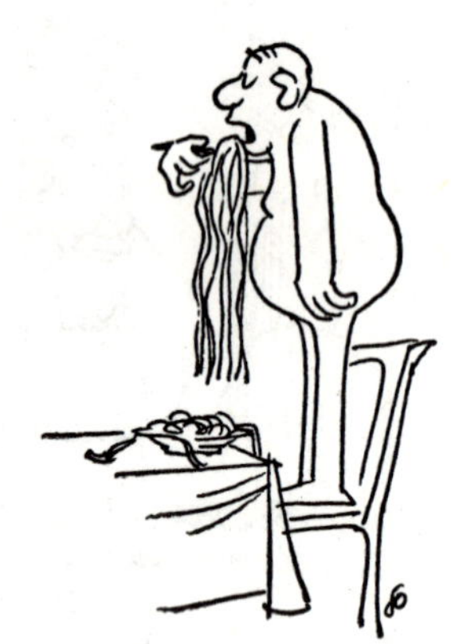

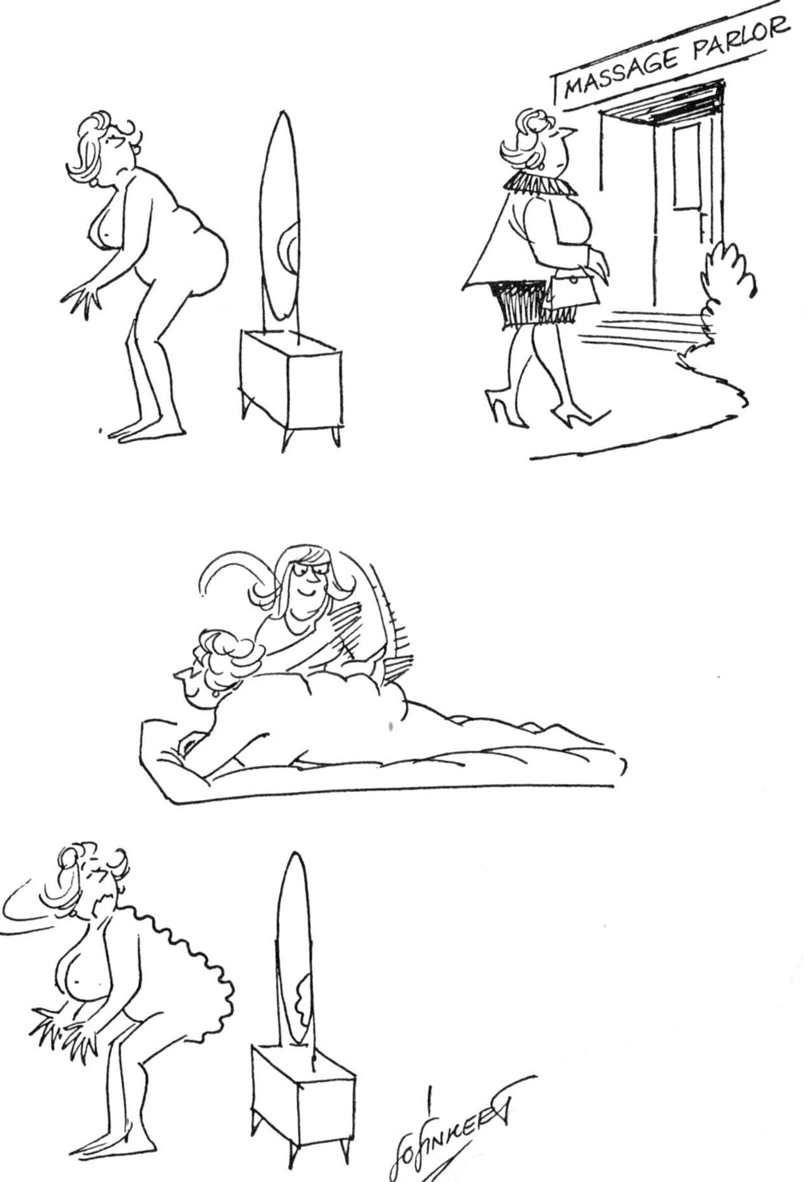
MASSAGE PARLOR
SOFINKERT

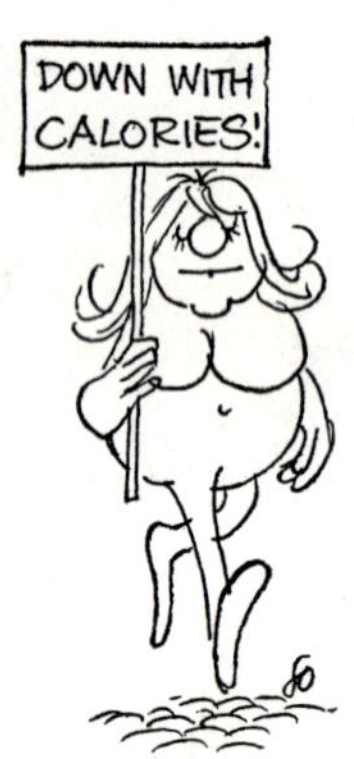
DOWN WITH
CALORIES!

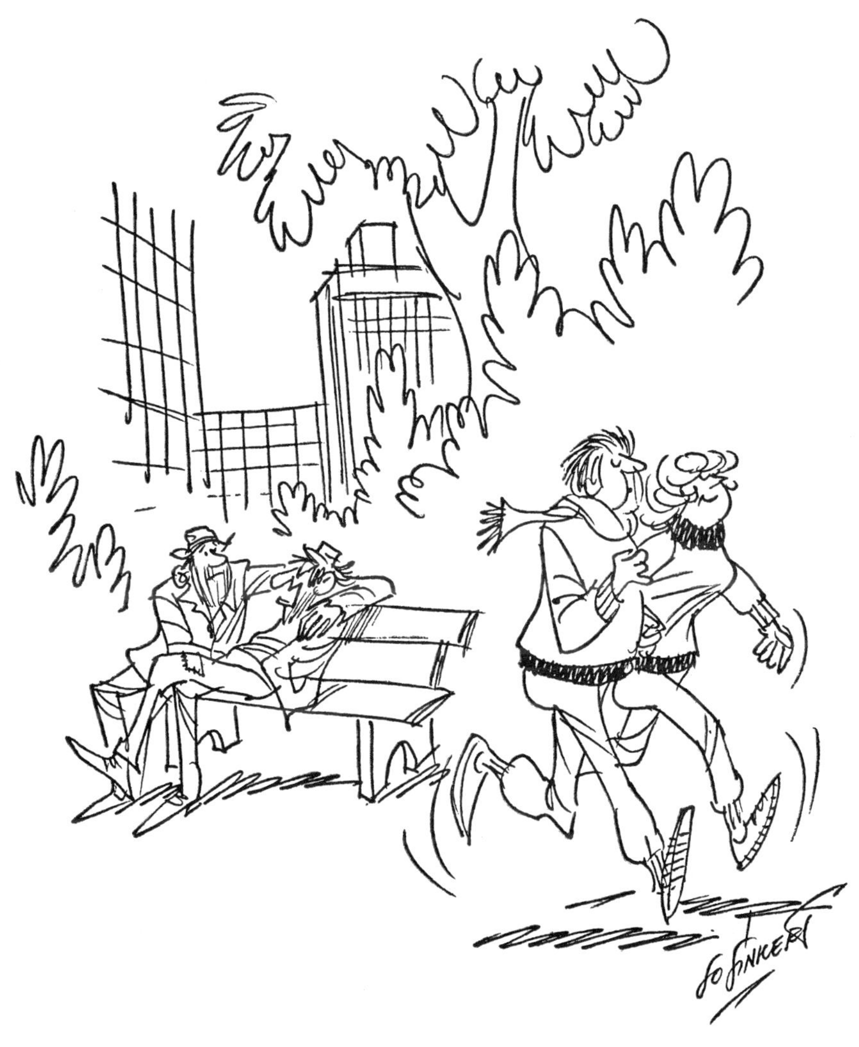

"I'M NOT GOING TO GET INVOLVED IN JOGGING UNTIL I SEE WHETHER IT'S HERE TO STAY."

I'M SO FULL OF GAS THAT THE DOCTOR WON'T GIVE ME ACUPUNCTURE.

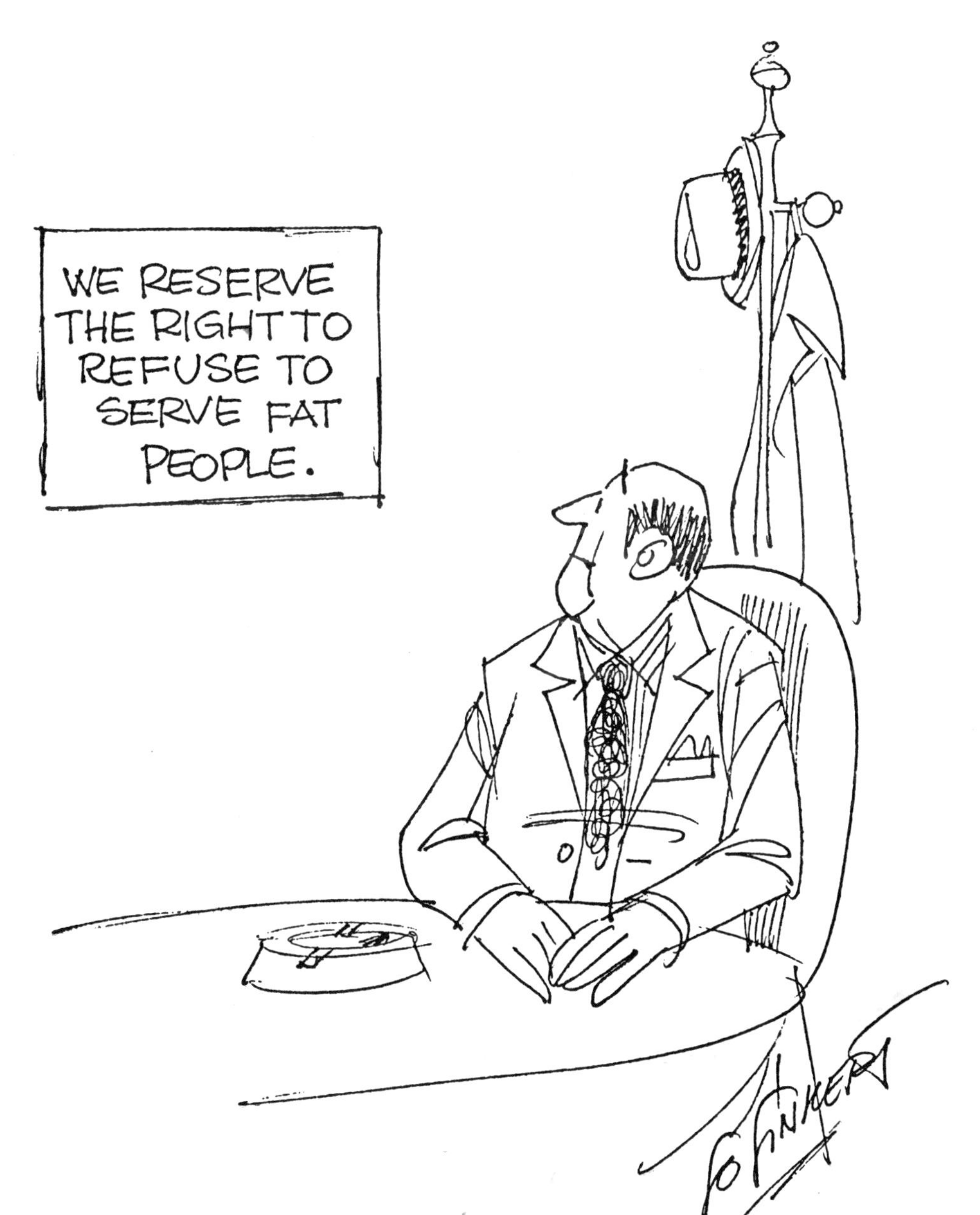
WE RESERVE
THE RIGHT TO
REFUSE TO
SERVE FAT
PEOPLE.

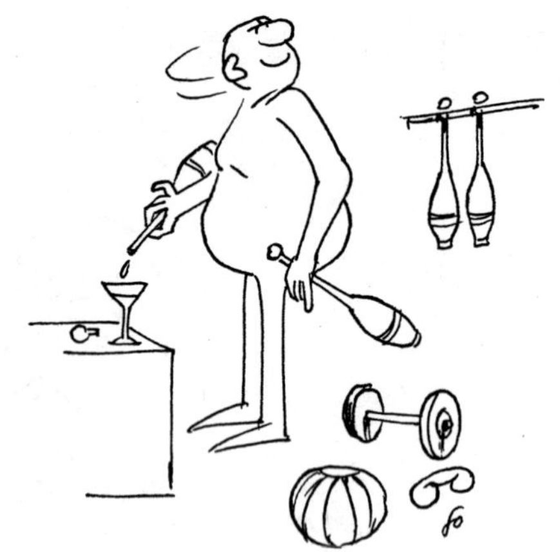

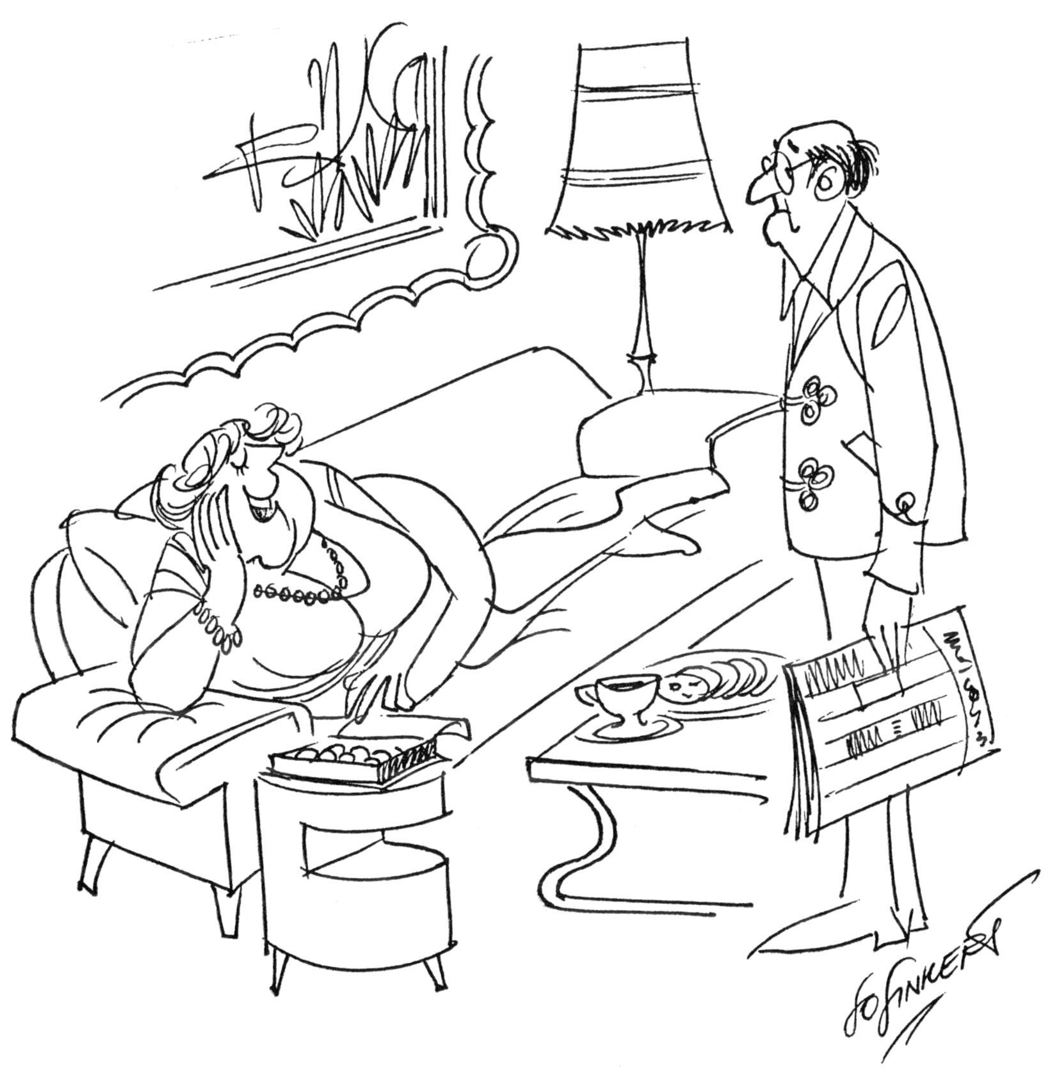

"I VE FOUND THE NICEST NEW DOCTOR, HE'S GOT A METABOLISM PROBLEM TOO."

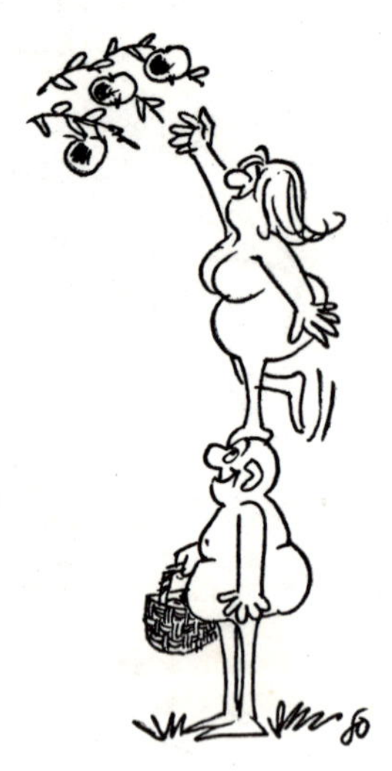

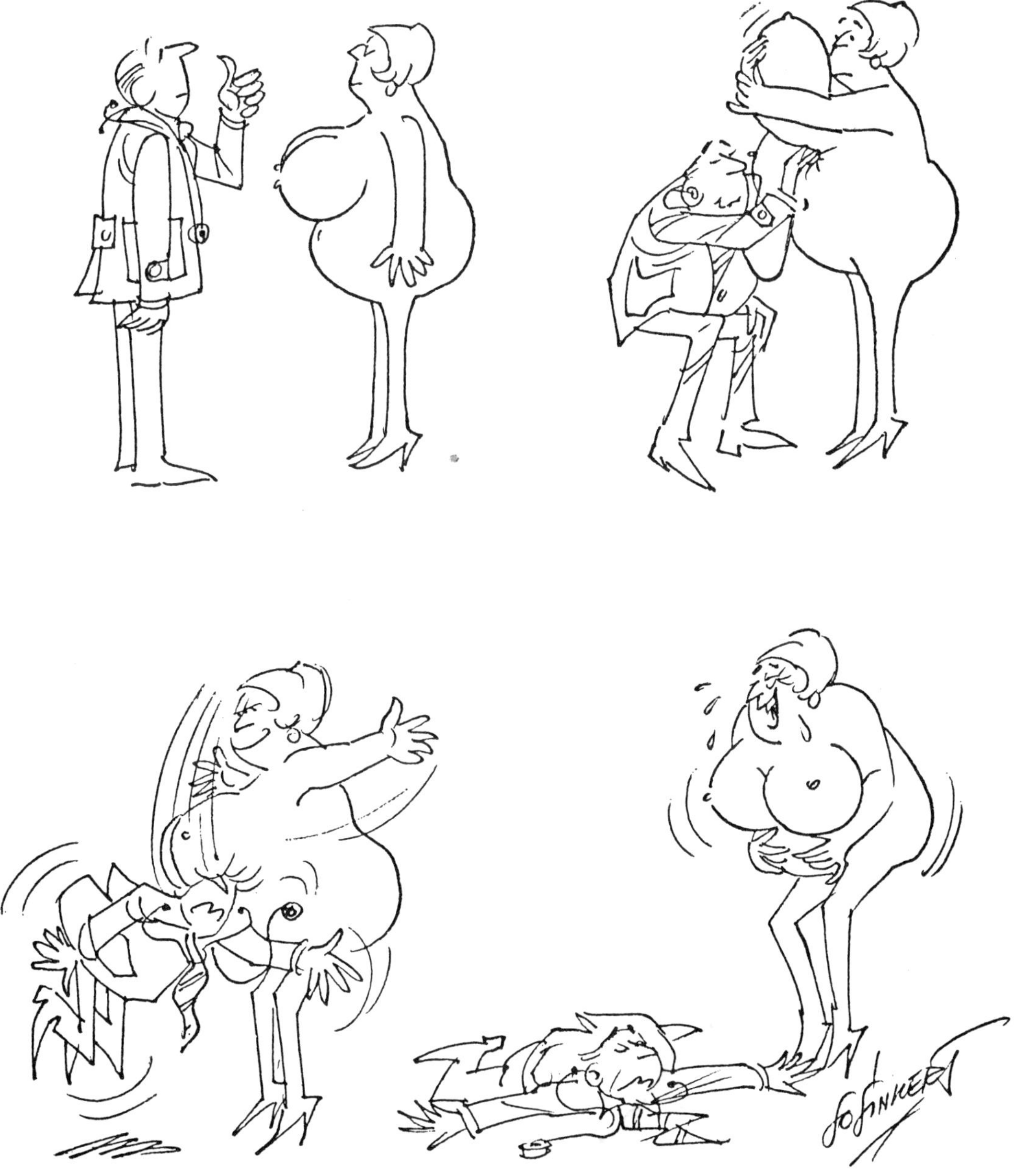

IF A WINE DRINKER
IS CALLED A WINO,
WHY ISN'T A RYE DRINKER
CALLED A RHINO?

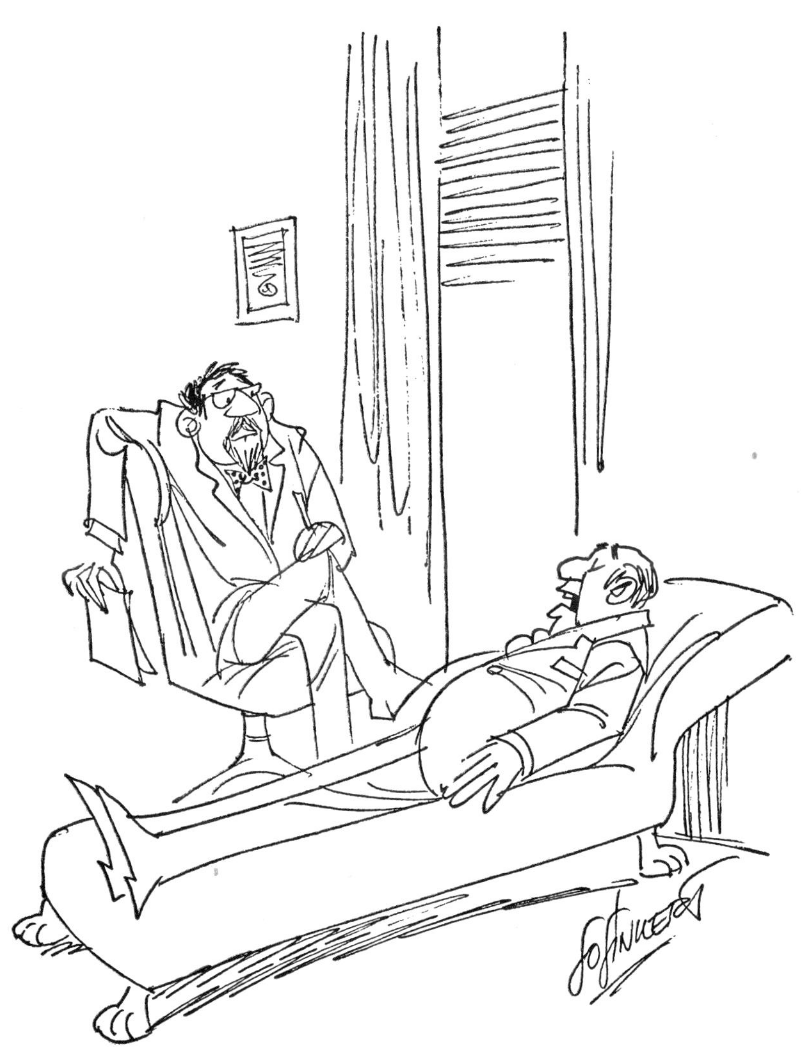

"I'M NOT INTERESTED IN LOSING WEIGHT, I'M INTERESTED IN LOSING MY GUILT FEELING OVER NOT LOSING WEIGHT."

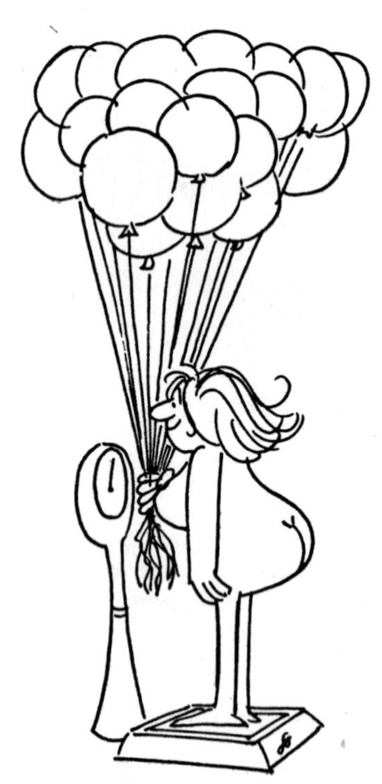

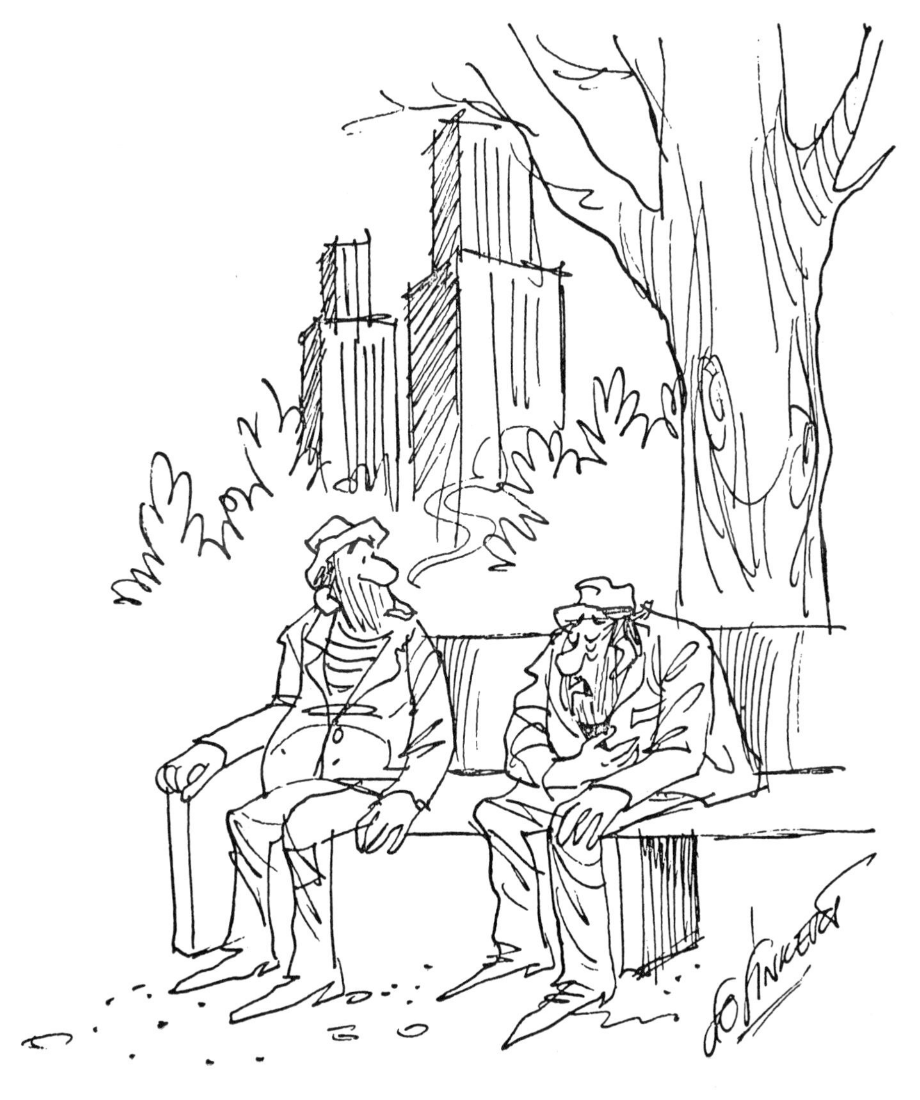

"I THINK I ATE SOMETHING FRESH."

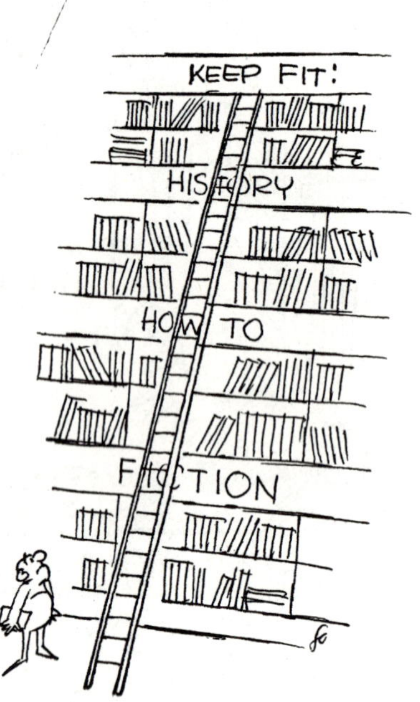
KEEP FIT!
HISTORY
HOW TO
FICTION

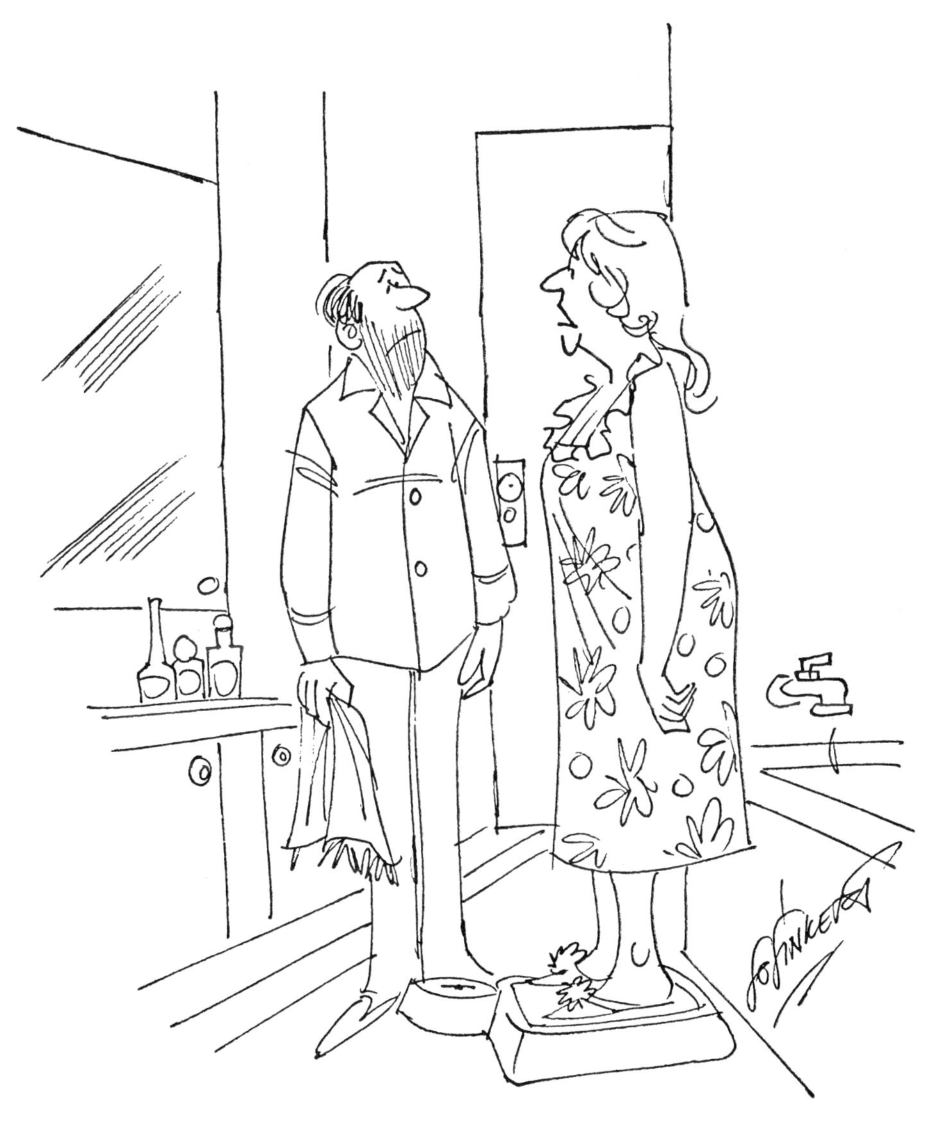

" IT'S TIMES LIKE THIS I WISH I WAS A BORN LOSER."

EAT FISH - LIVE LONGER
EAT OYSTERS - LOVE LONGER

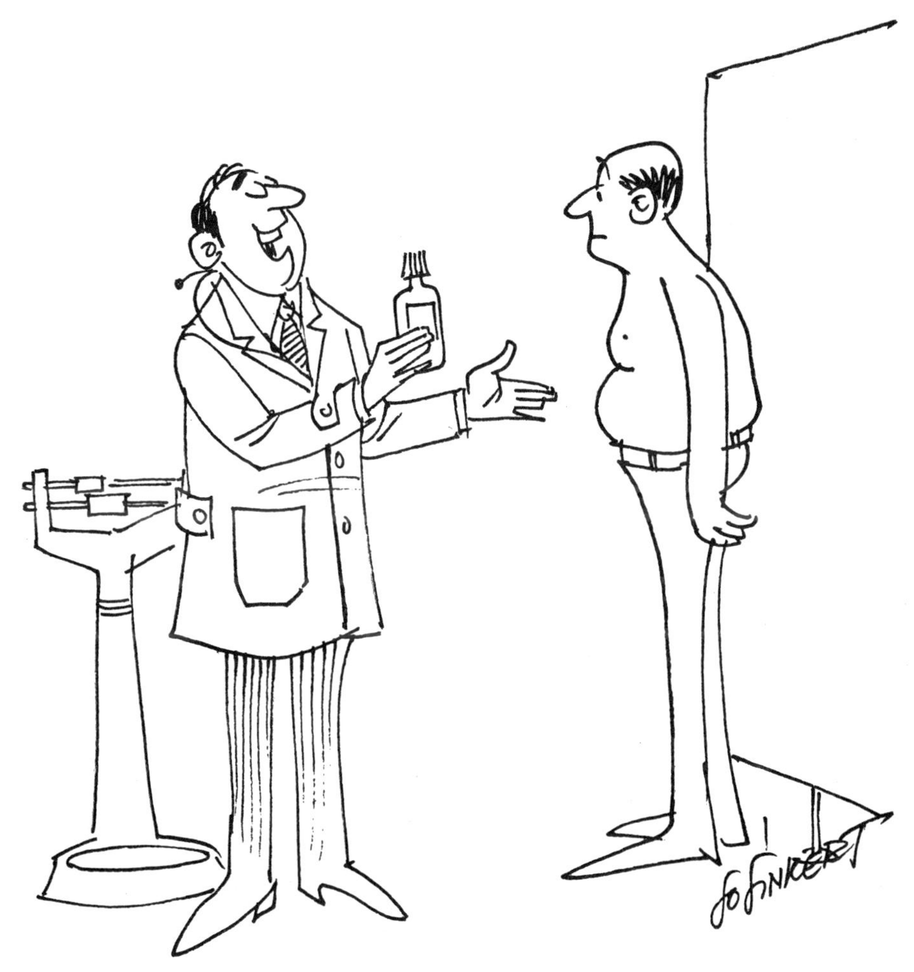

" TAKE ONE SPOONFUL AFTER EACH MEAL..
ER... BY THE WAY, HOW
ARE YOU AT THE 100 YARD DASH? "

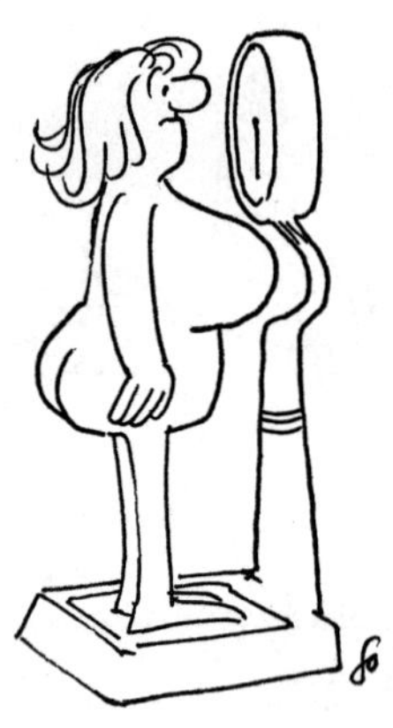

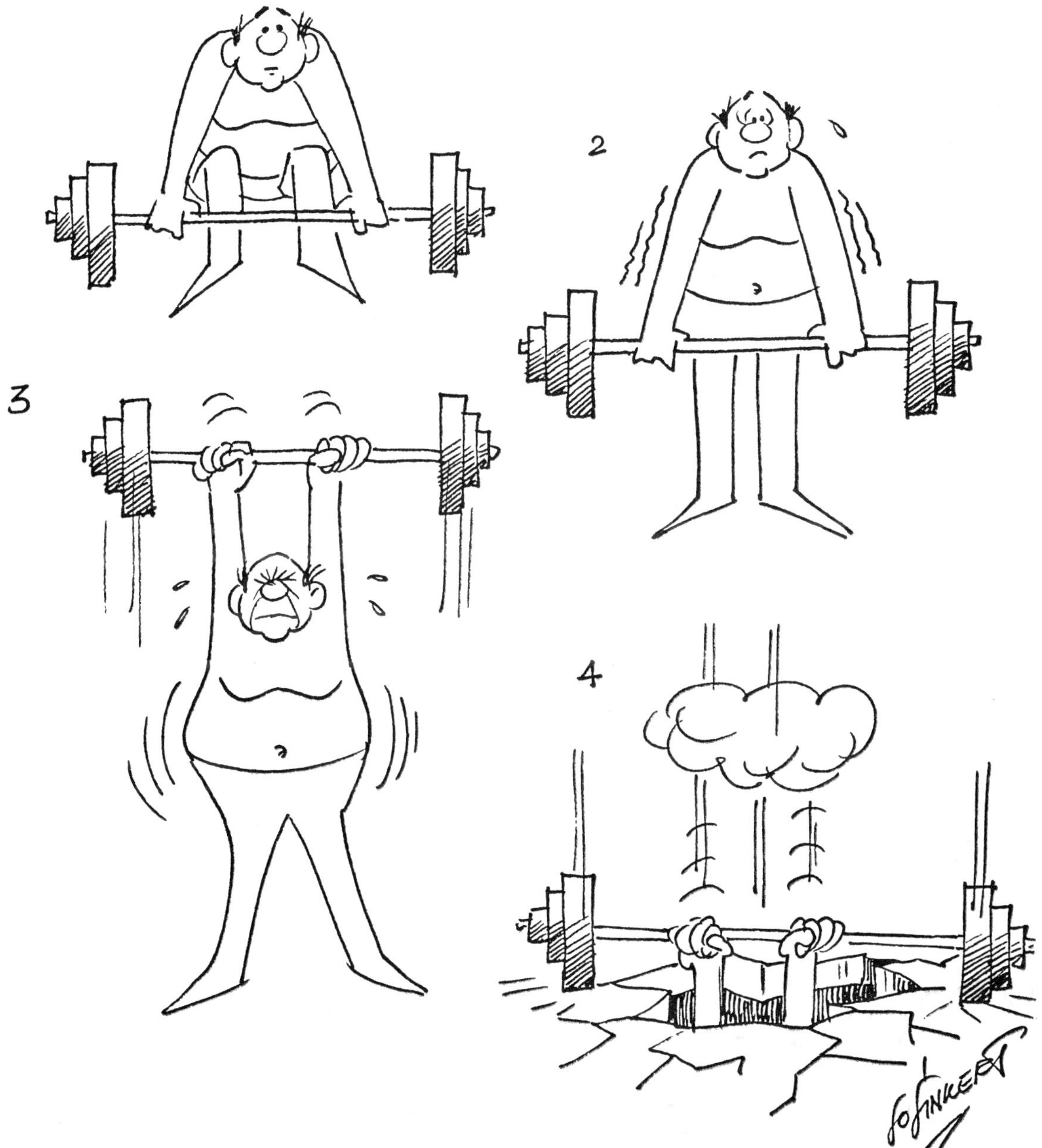
2
3
4

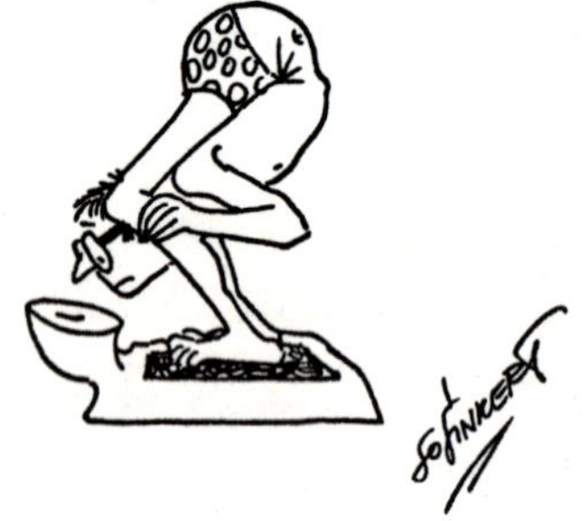

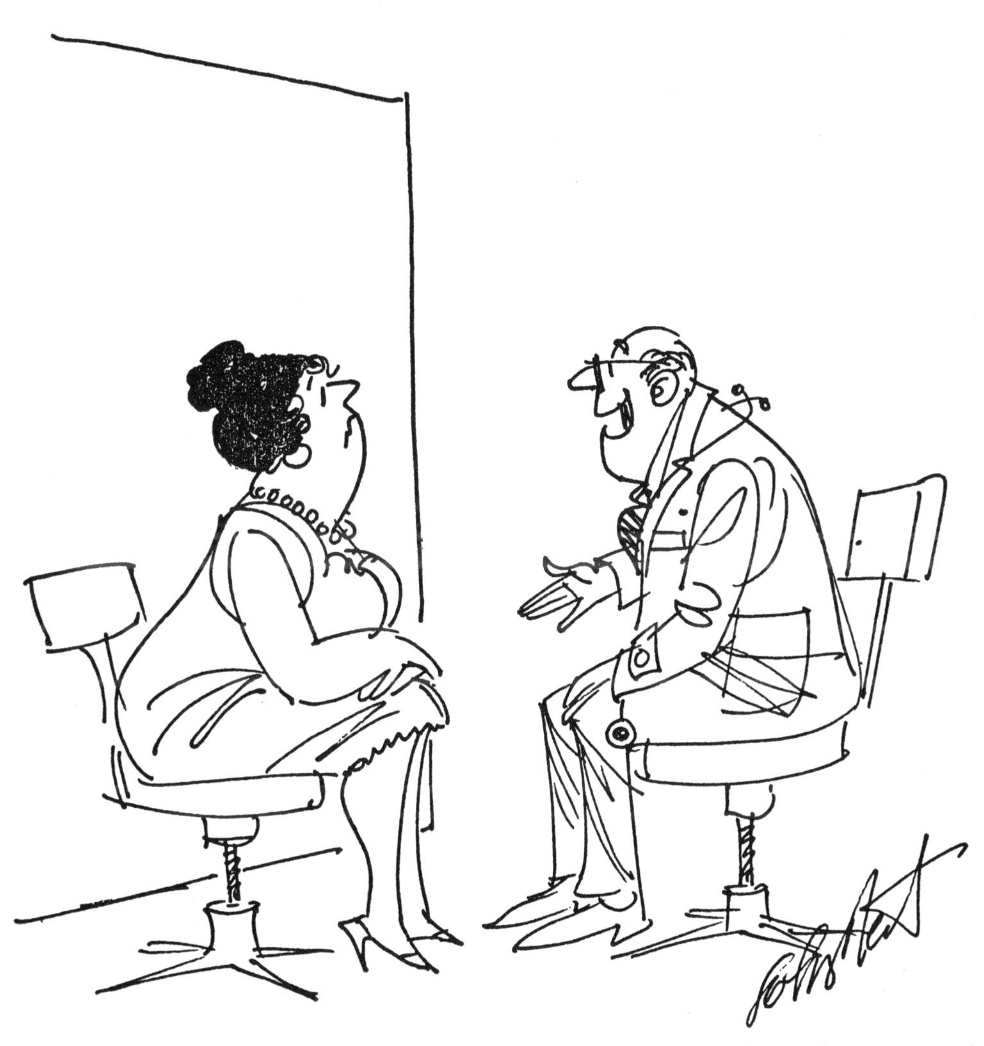

"GOOD NEWS MS. JASBEC, YOU CAN HAVE ALL YOU WANT OF ANYTHING YOU CAN'T STAND."

IF SOMEONE WOULD INVENT A FAT-DONATION, THE WORLD WOULD BE FULL OF BIG SPENDERS.

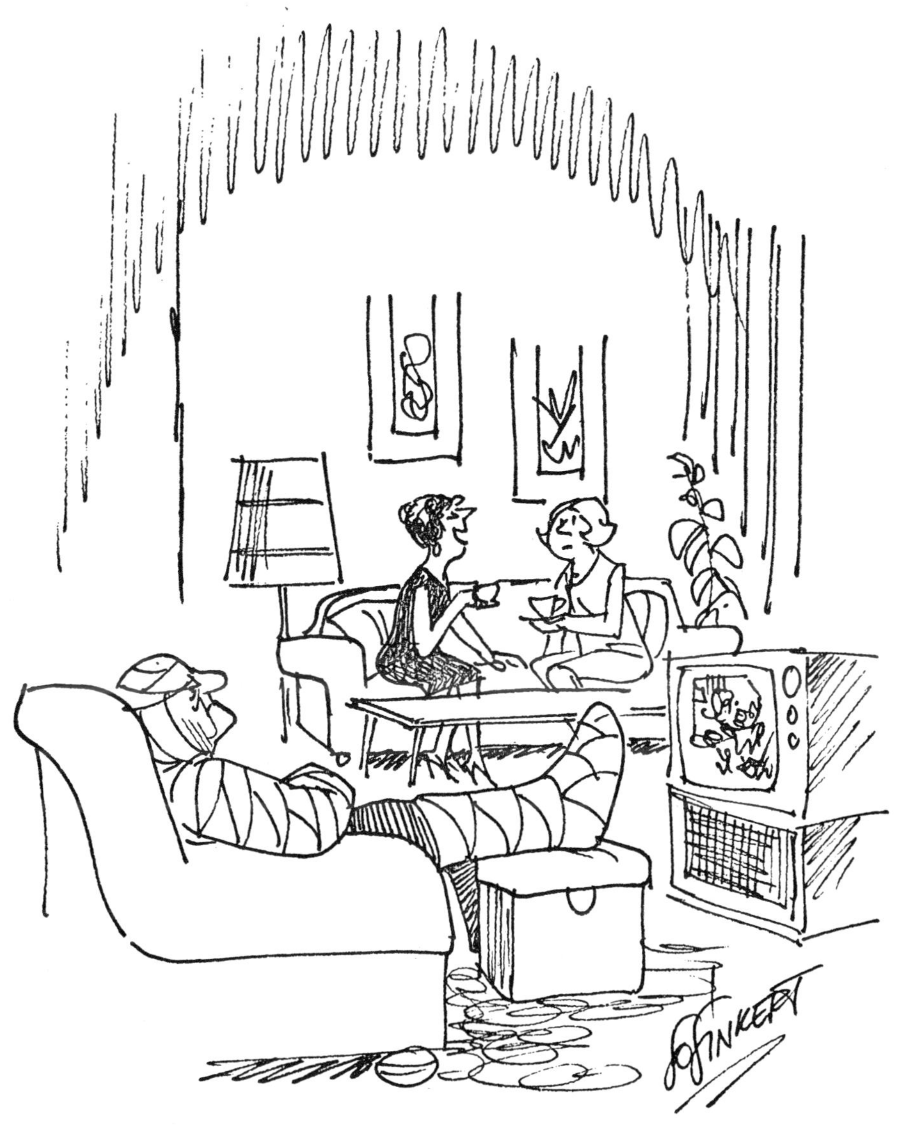

" WELL, FIRST HE SLIPPED WHILE JOGGING, THEN HE FELL OFF HIS EXERCISE MACHINE, AND FINALLY SOMEONE IN HIS FITNESS CLASS DROPPED SOME BARBELLS ON HIS HEAD . . ."

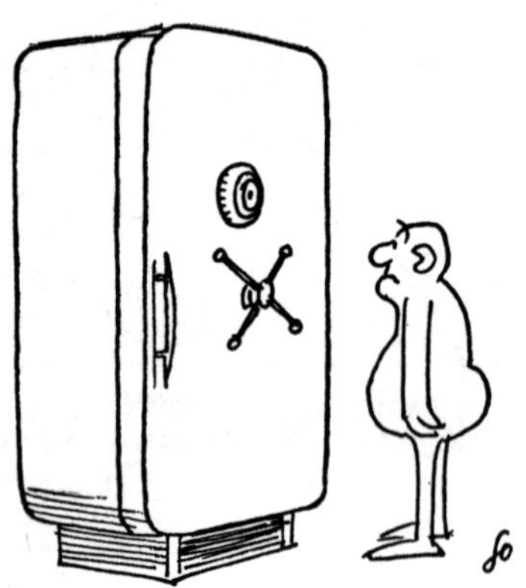

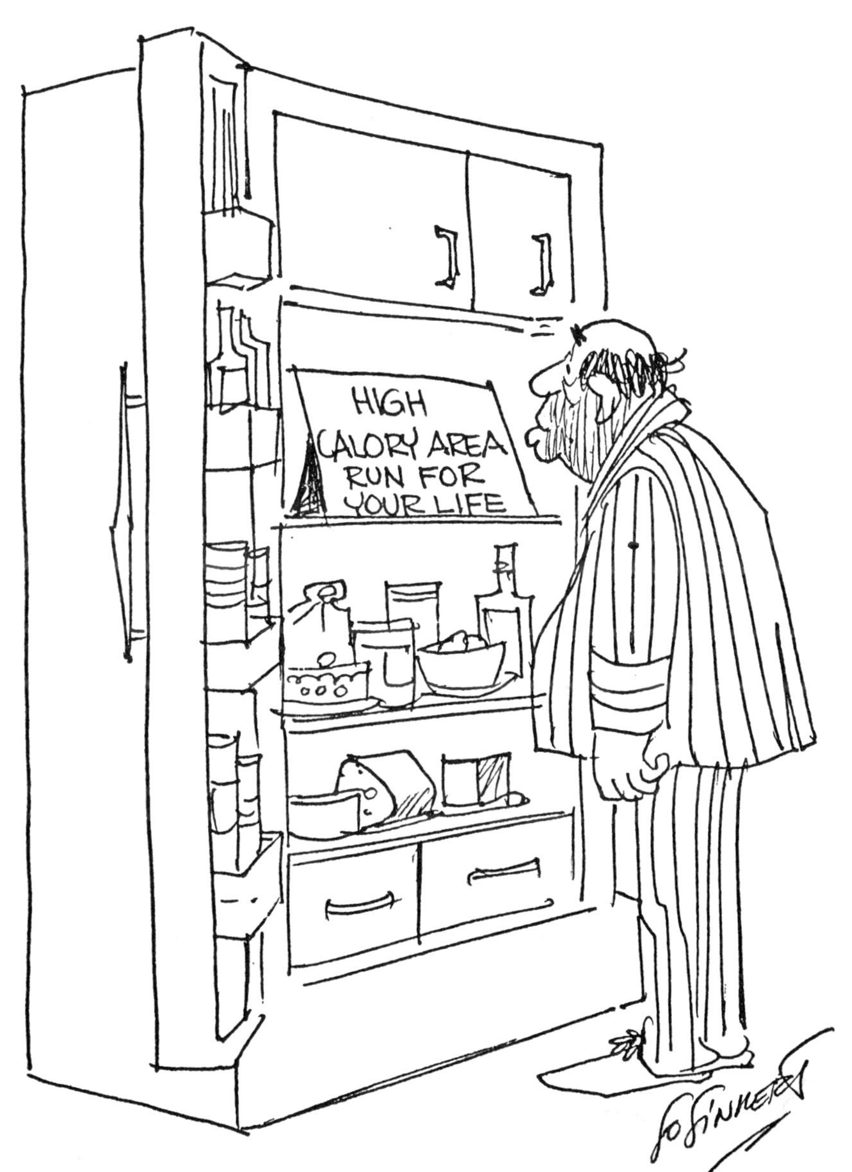
HIGH
CALORY AREA
RUN FOR
YOUR LIFE

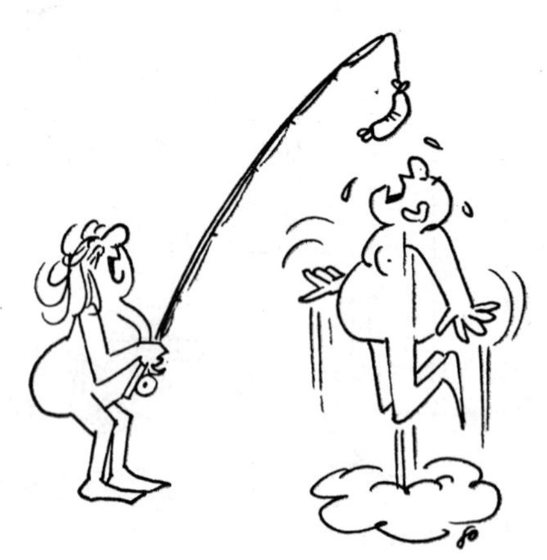

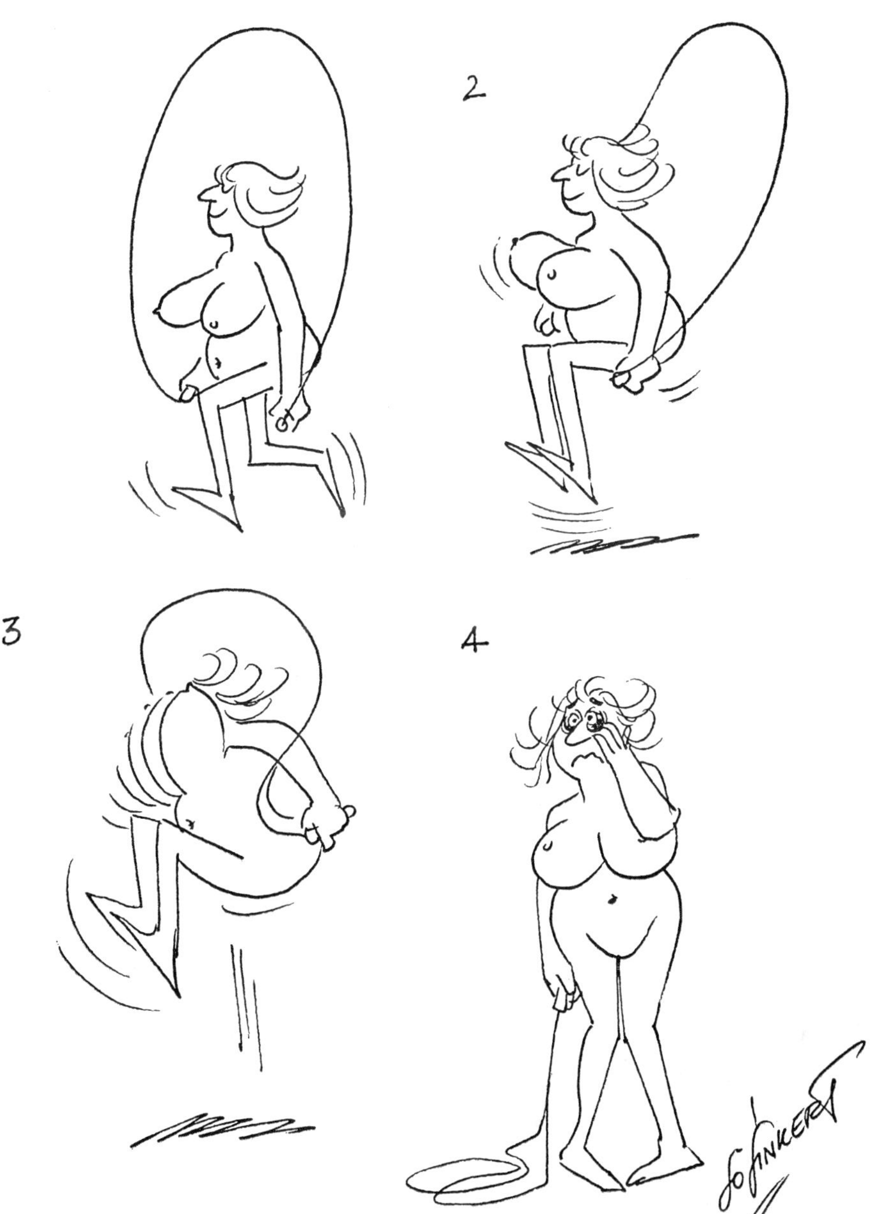
2
3
4

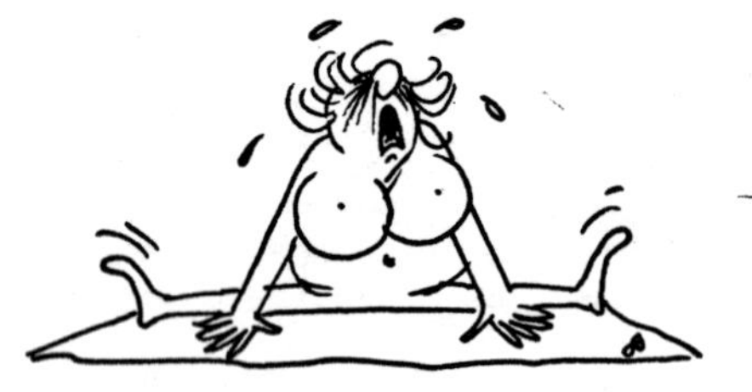

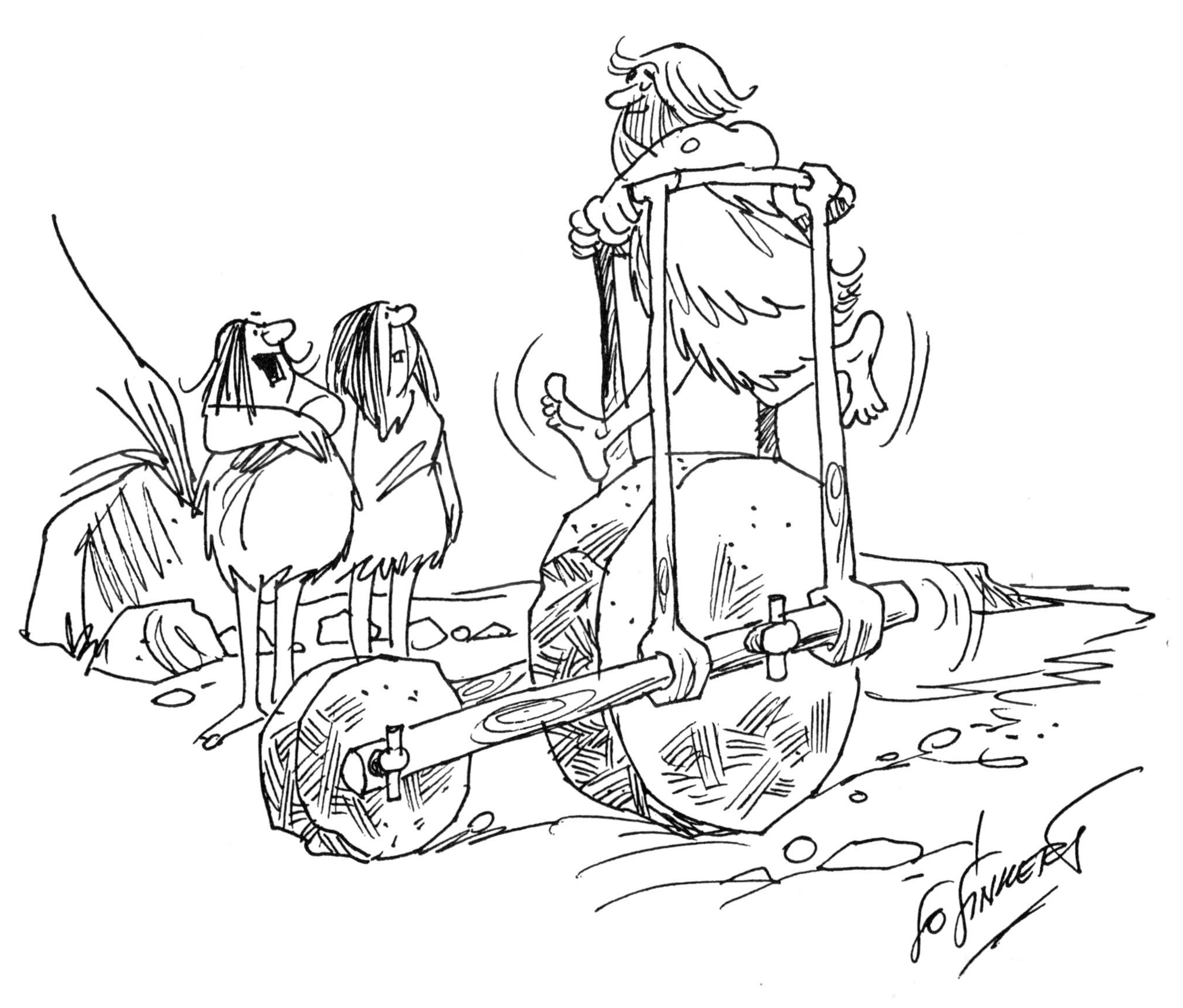

"HE SAYS IT BEATS WALKING."

A SURE WAY TO LOSE WEIGHT: MIX RUM AND PRUNE JUICE – IT'S CALLED A RUM RUNNER.

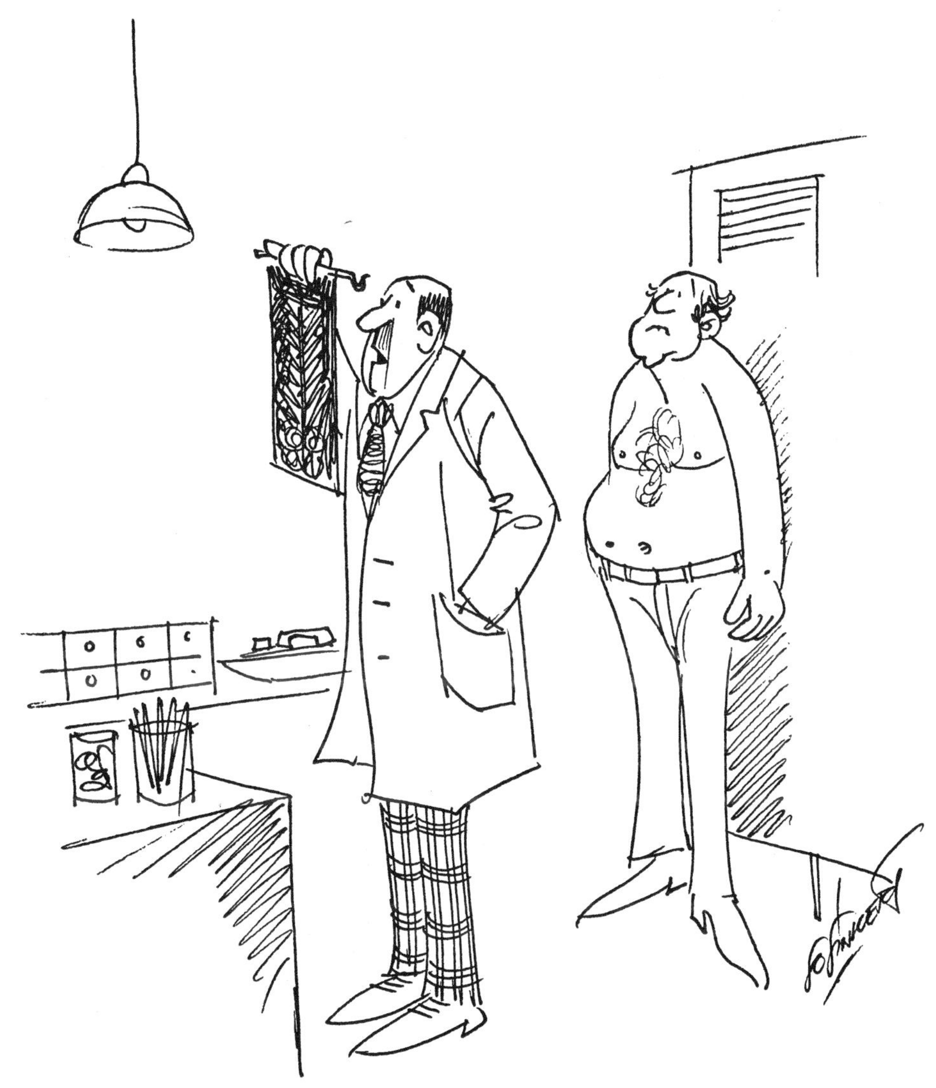

"YOU NEED MORE EXERCISE; YOUR GALLSTONES ARE GATHERING MOSS."

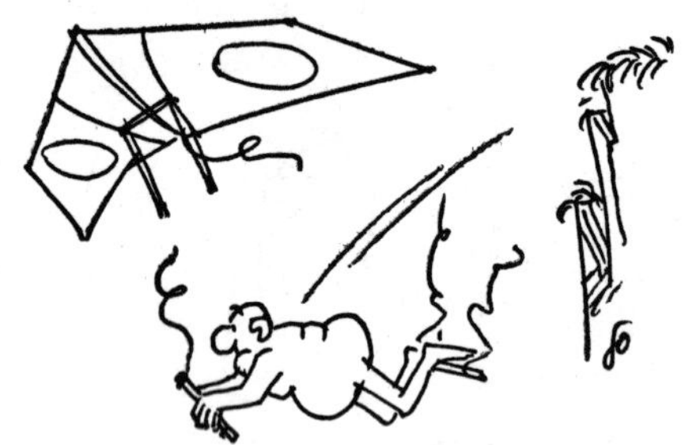

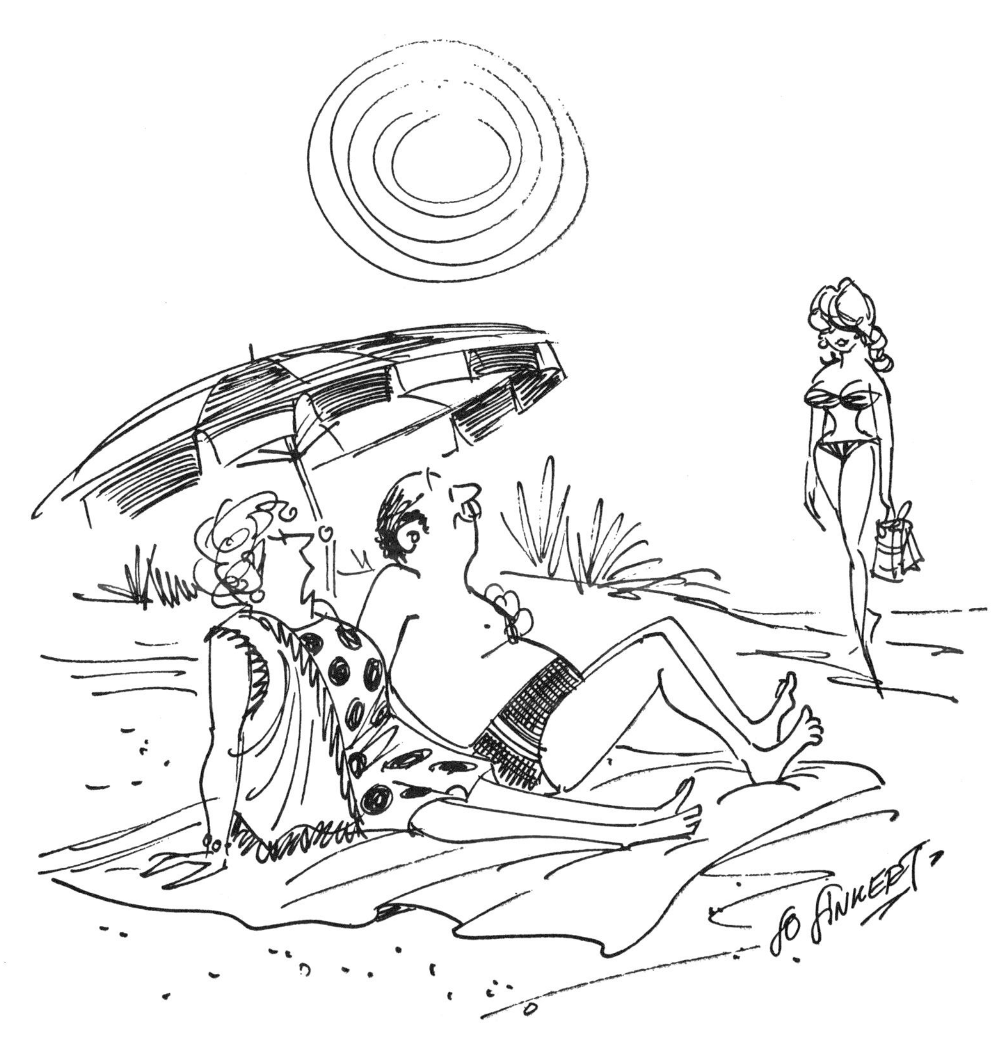

YOU NEVER BREATHE THAT WAY WHEN I WEAR MY BIKINI."

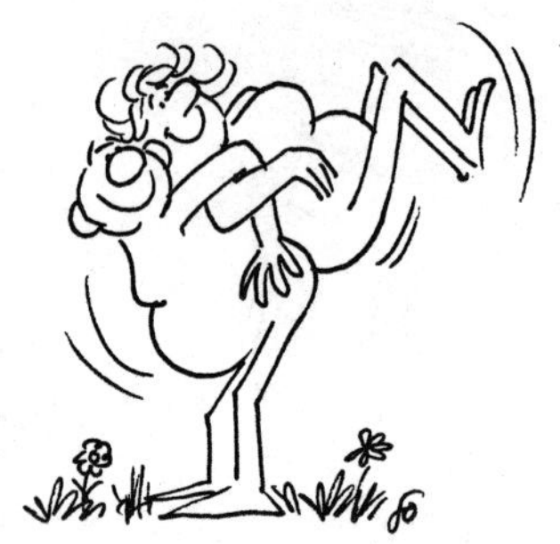

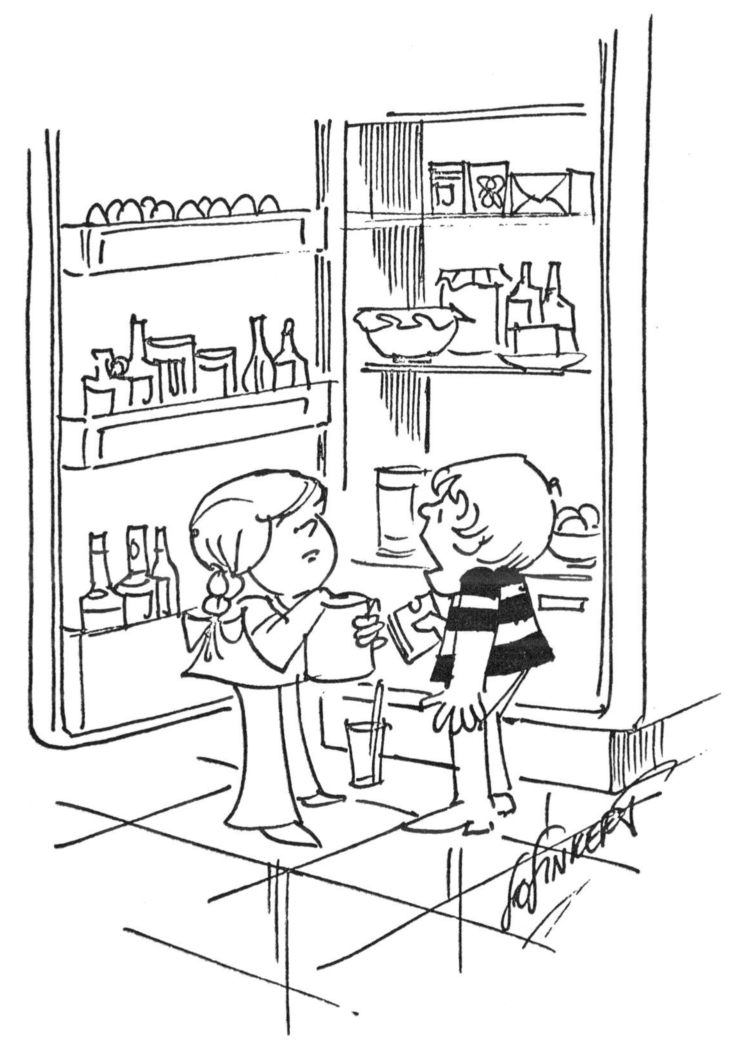

" DON'T EAT A DILL PICKLE WITH IT-
THAT MADE MOM FAT."

BEFORE YOU KNOW IT,
OVERWEIGHT SNACKS
UP ON YOU.

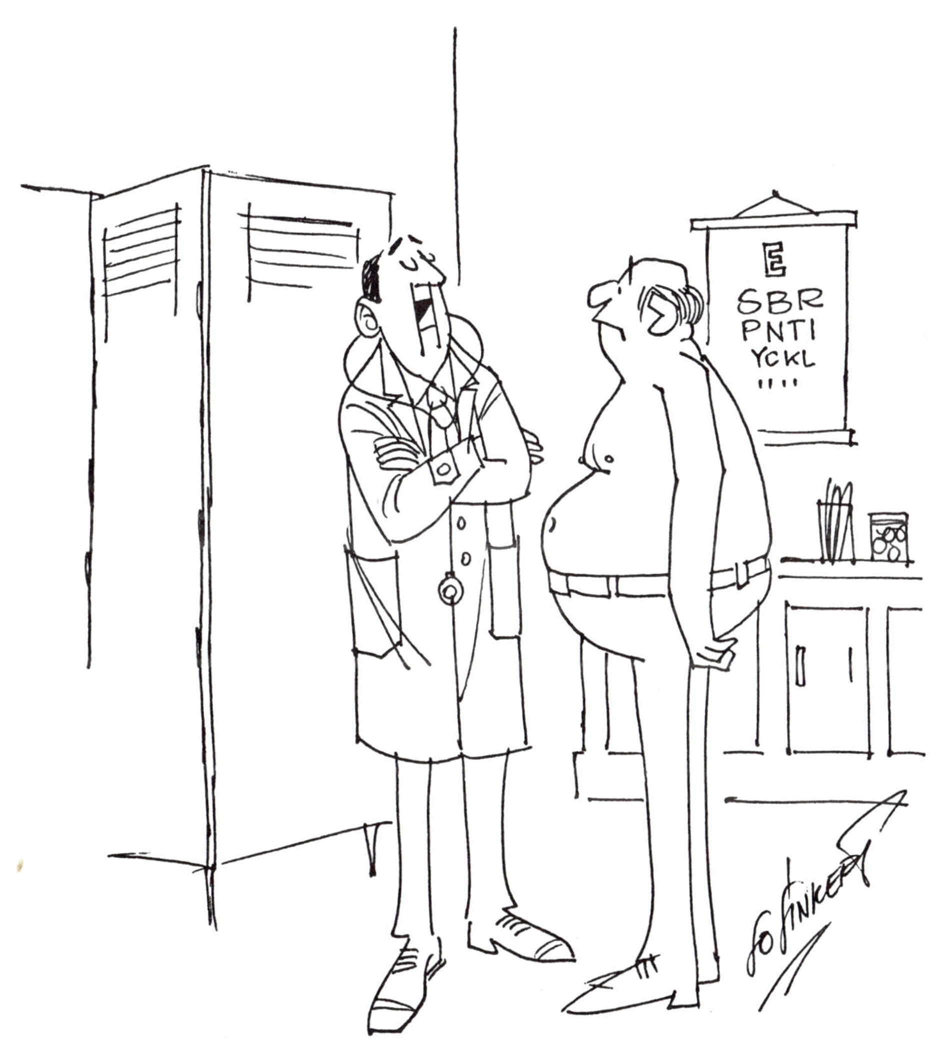

" REGARDLESS OF THE GOVERNMENT'S PROGRAM, THEY CAN'T DO ANYTHING FOR YOUR TYPE INFLATION."

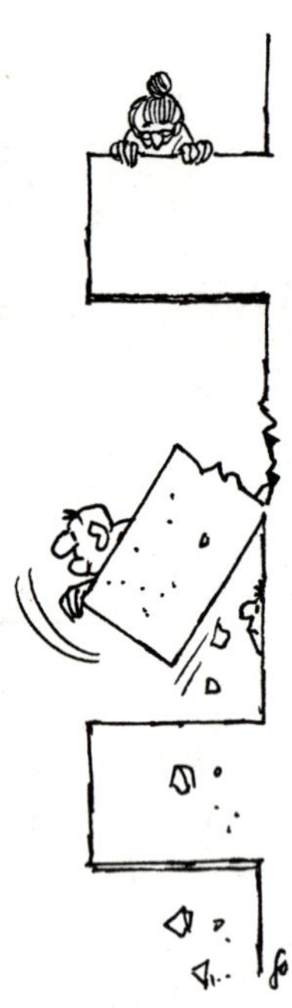

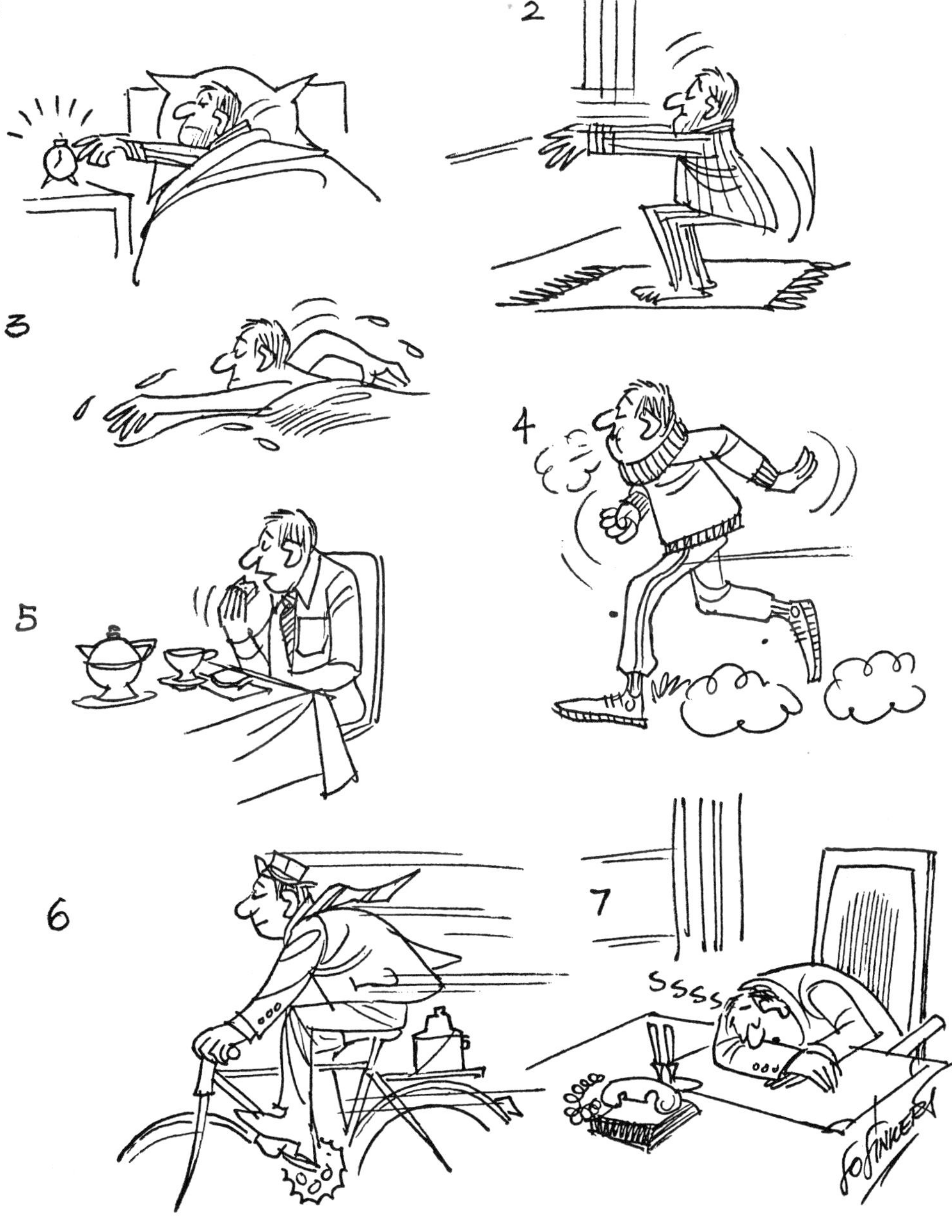
1
2
3
4
5
6
7
SSSS

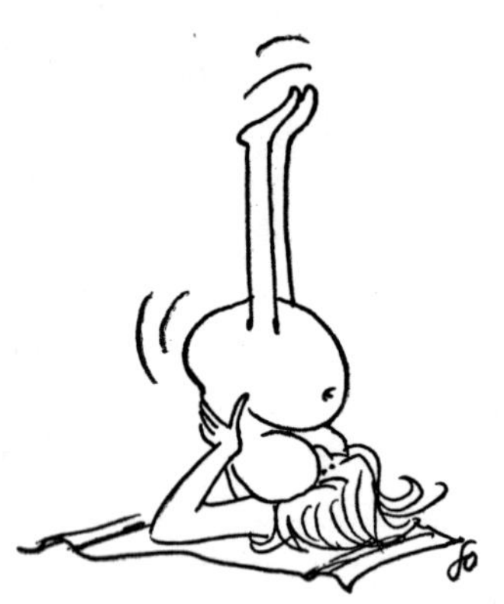

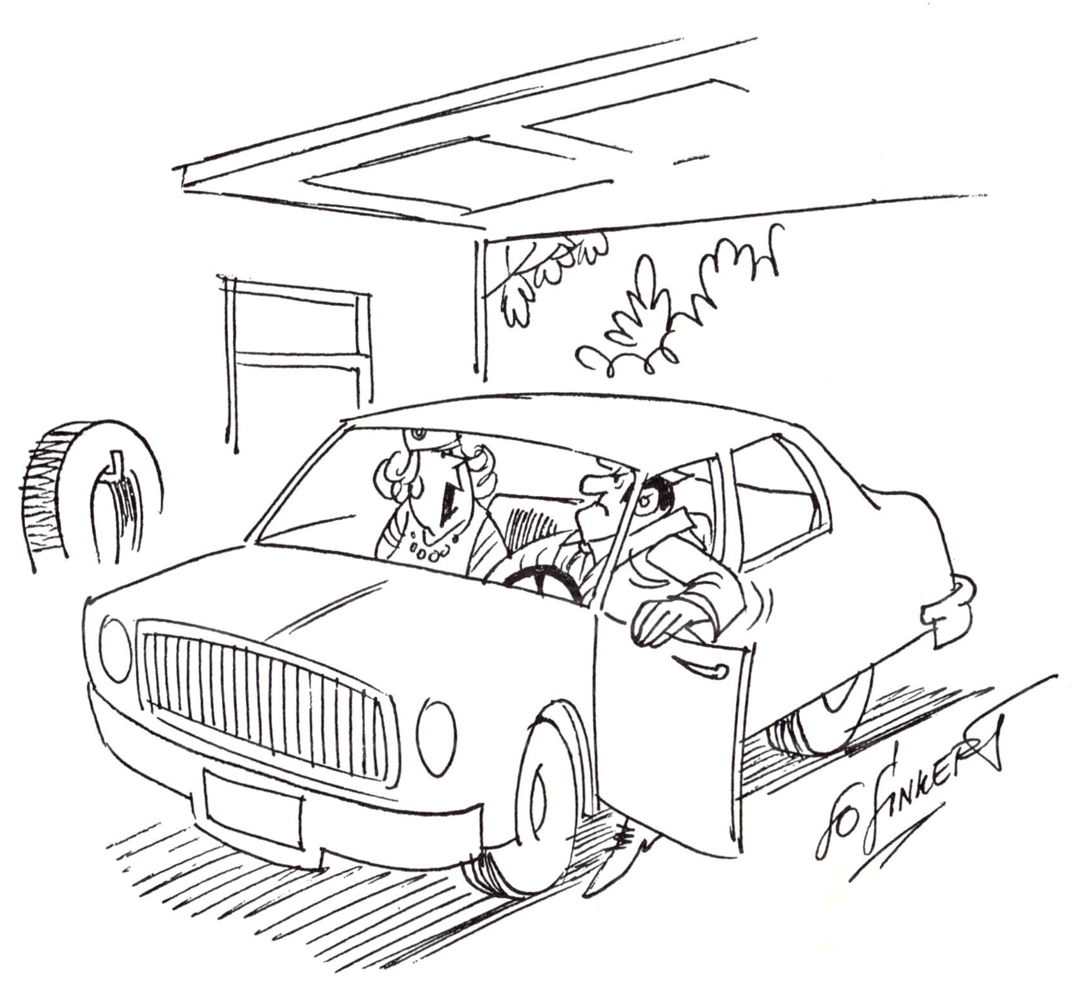

" JUST ONCE, HENRY, I WISH YOU'D GET INTO THE CAR WITHOUT BLOWING THE HORN."

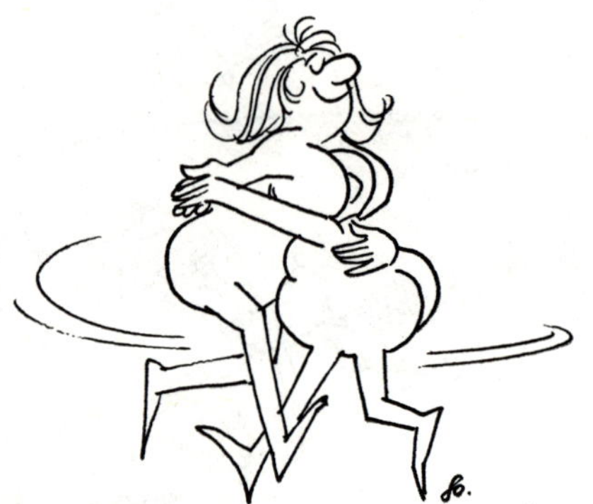

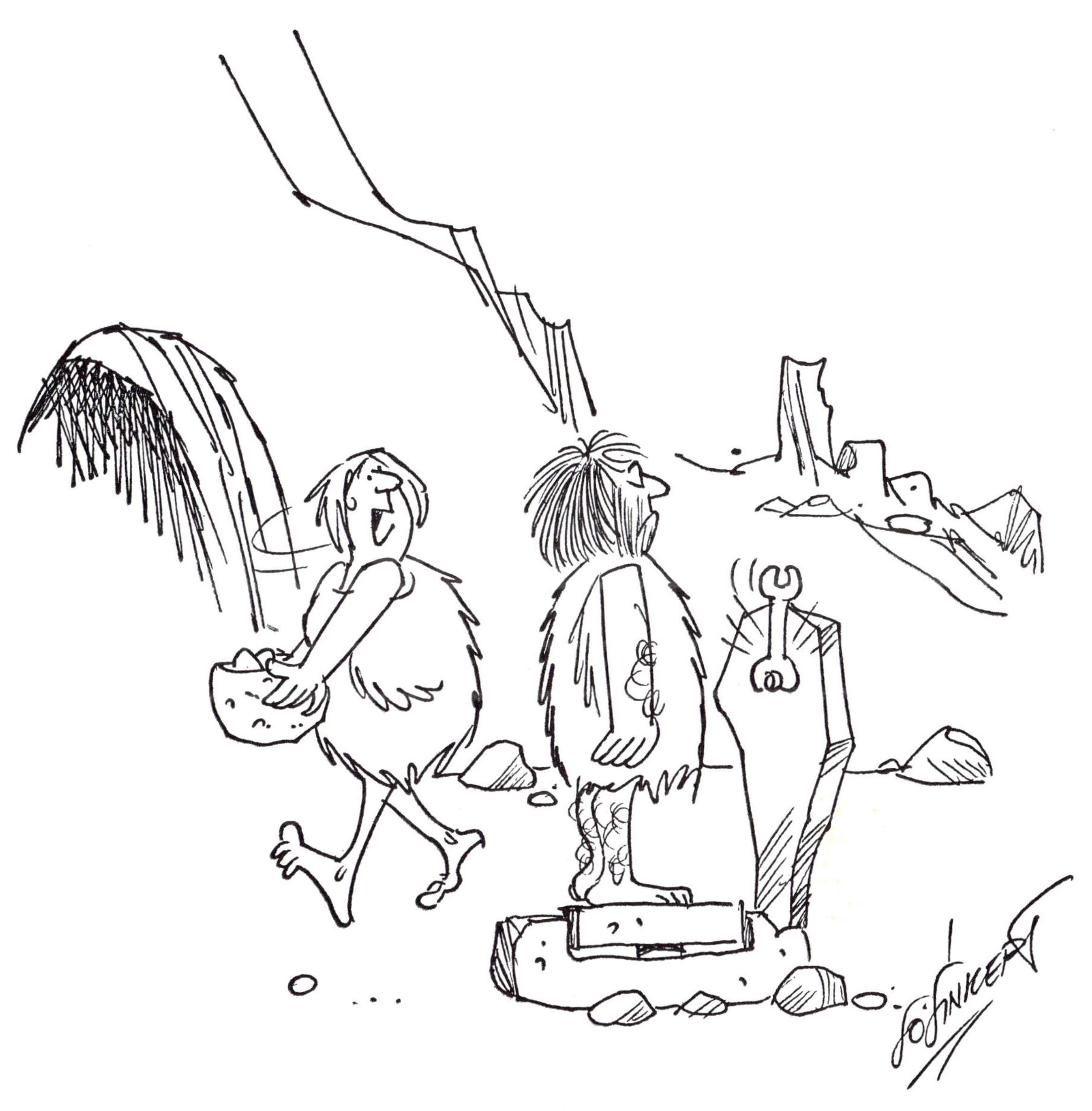

" WHO NEEDS IT? "

A BORN LOSER IS A
PERSON WHO GAINS
EVERY DAY.

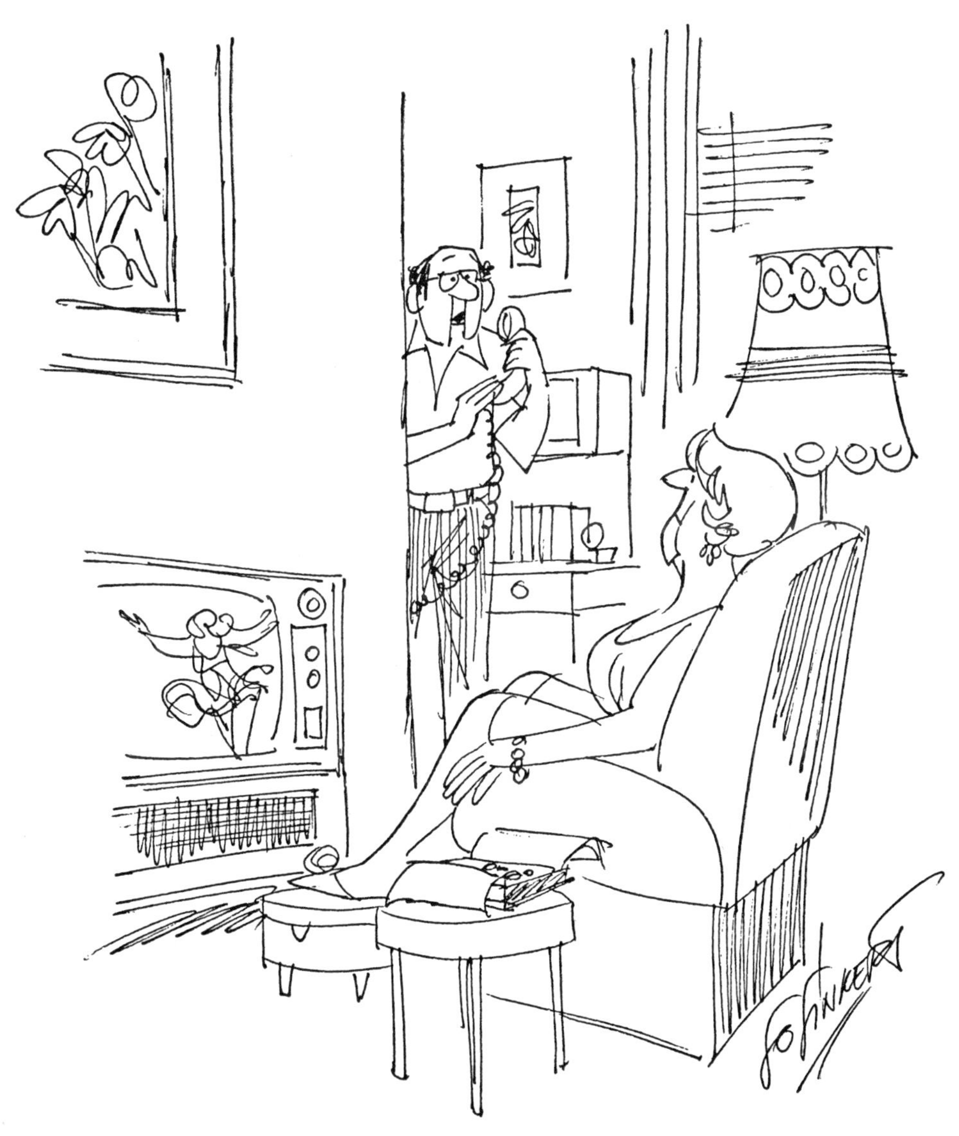

"IT'S THE HEALTH SPA, YOU'RE BEING RECALLED."

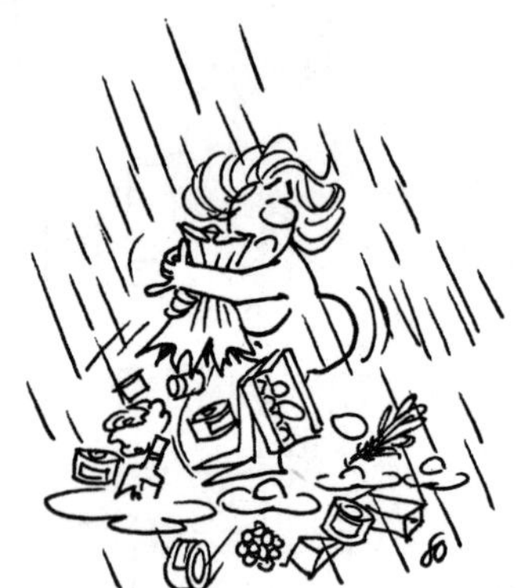

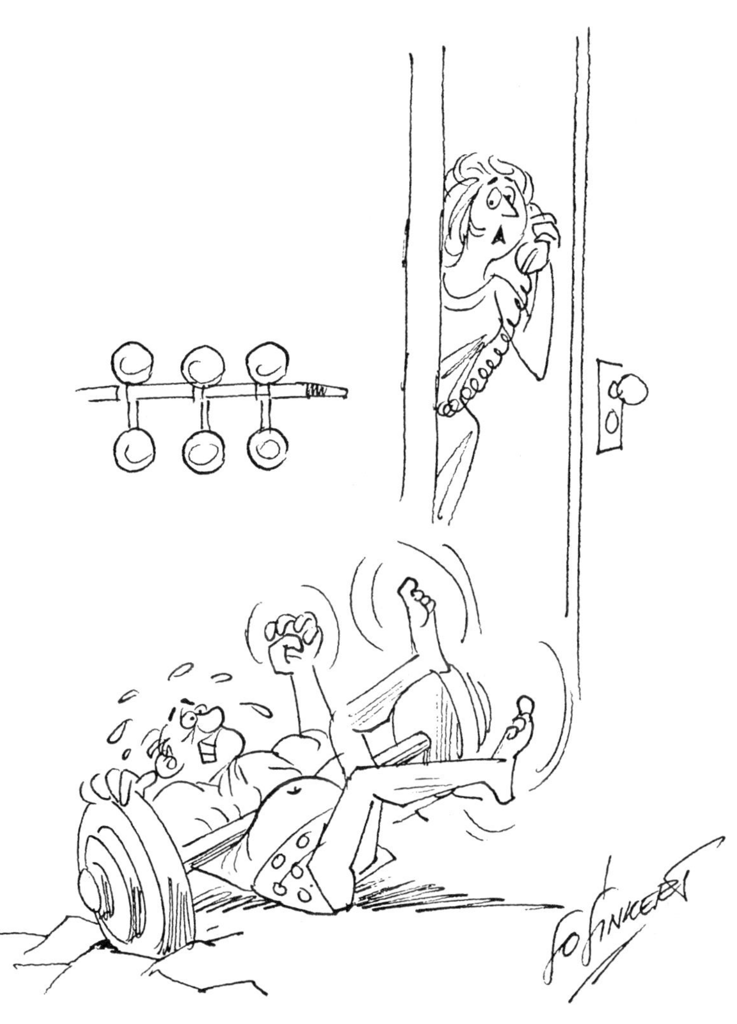

"HOLD ON A MINUTE, MARGE, ROGER WANTS ME TO GIVE HIM A HAND WITH SOMETHING!"

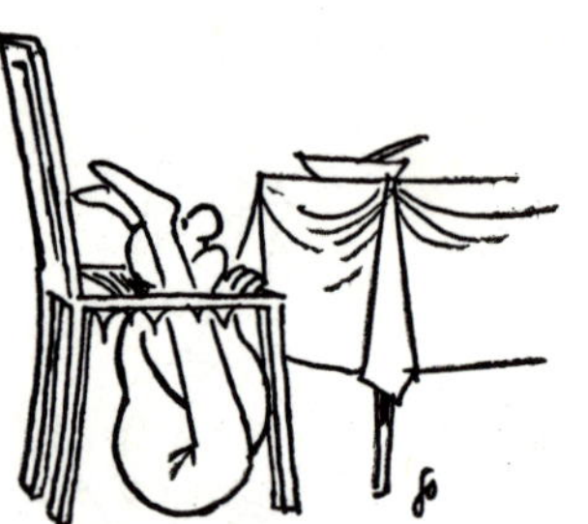

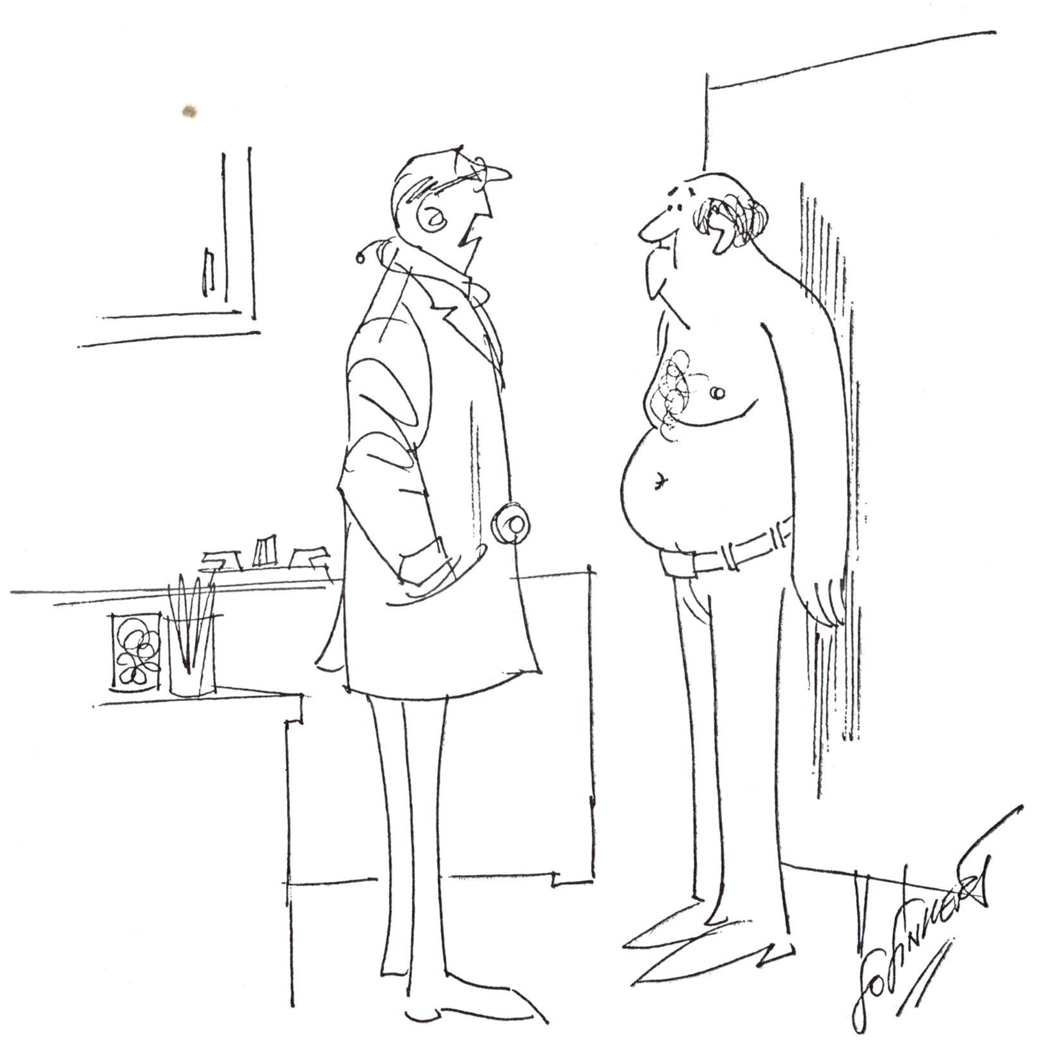

" NO WINE, MR CHAPPELL; NO WOMEN, AND IF YOU SHOULD FEEL LIKE SINGING YOU'D BETTER JUST HUM A LITTLE."

SWEETS WON'T HURT YOU
IF YOU WALK A MILE FOR
A CARAMEL.

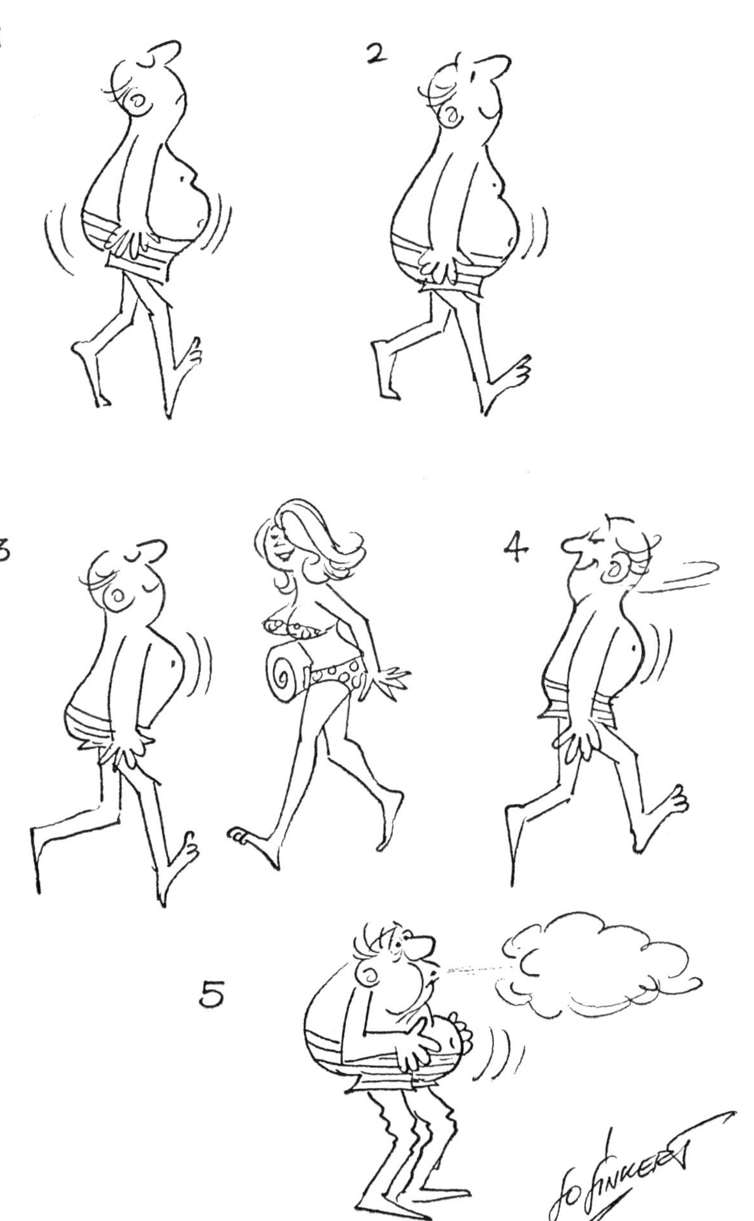
1
2
3
4
5

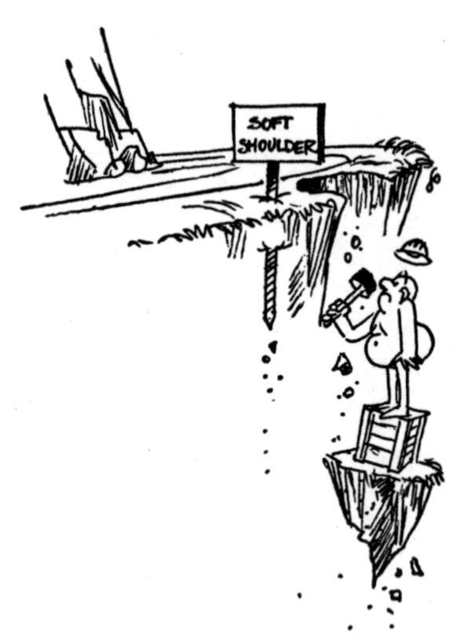
SOFT
SHOULDER

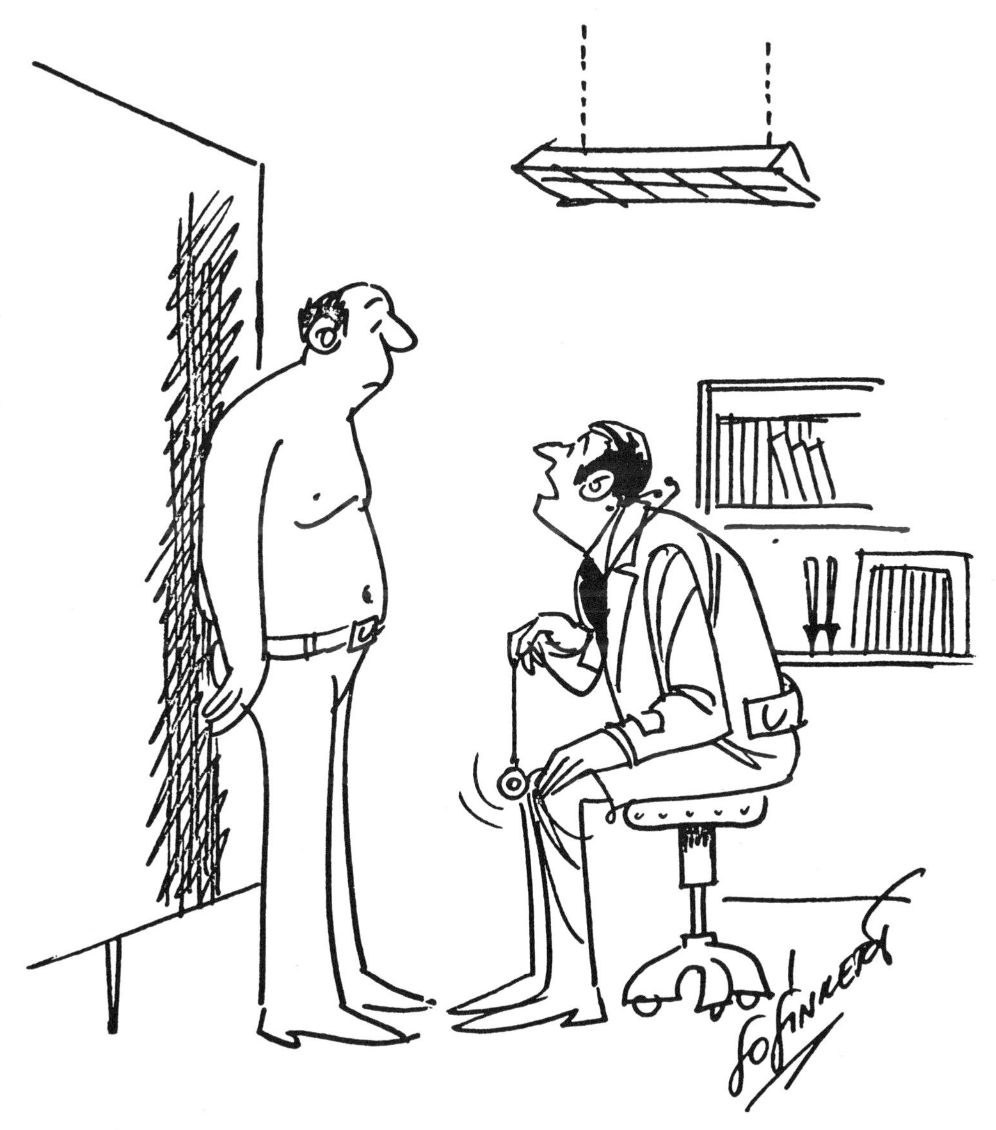

"THE SLOSHING OF THE BEER IS DROWNING OUT THE BEATING OF YOUR HEART."

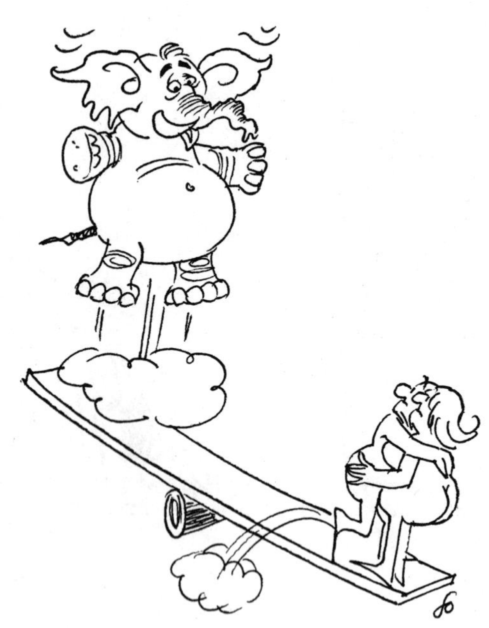

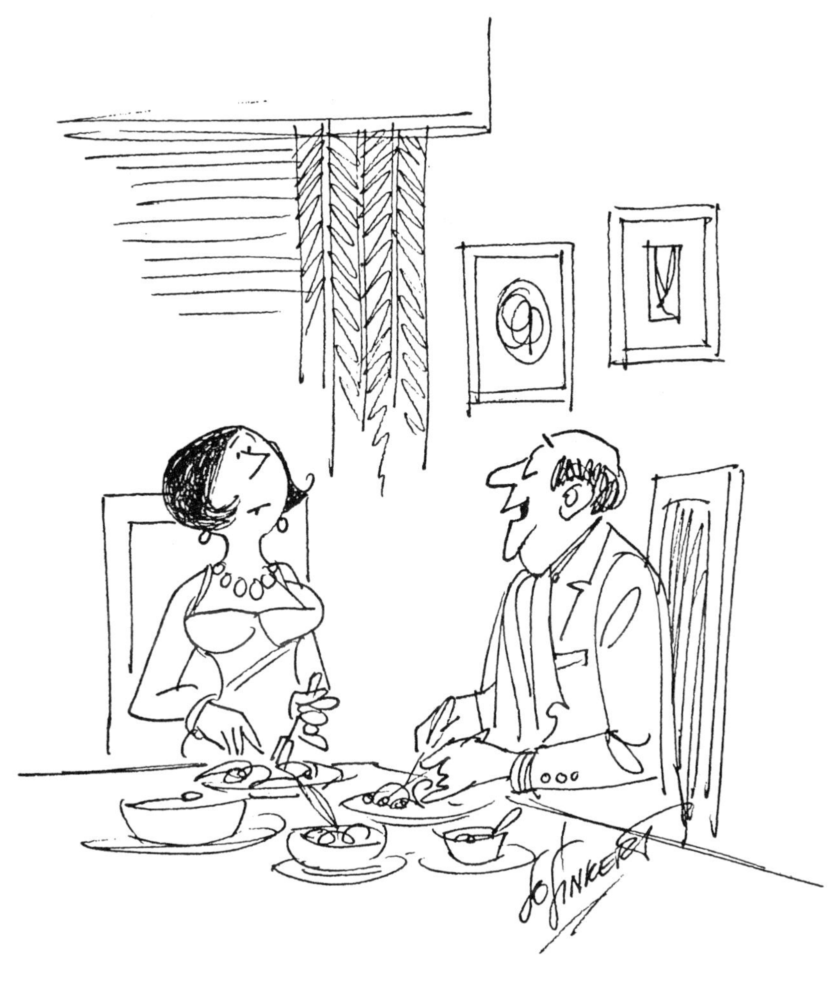

"I'M ON A SEAFOOD DIET. WHEN I SEE FOOD I EAT IT."

I WENT ON A WATER DIET
AND GAINED 12 LITERS

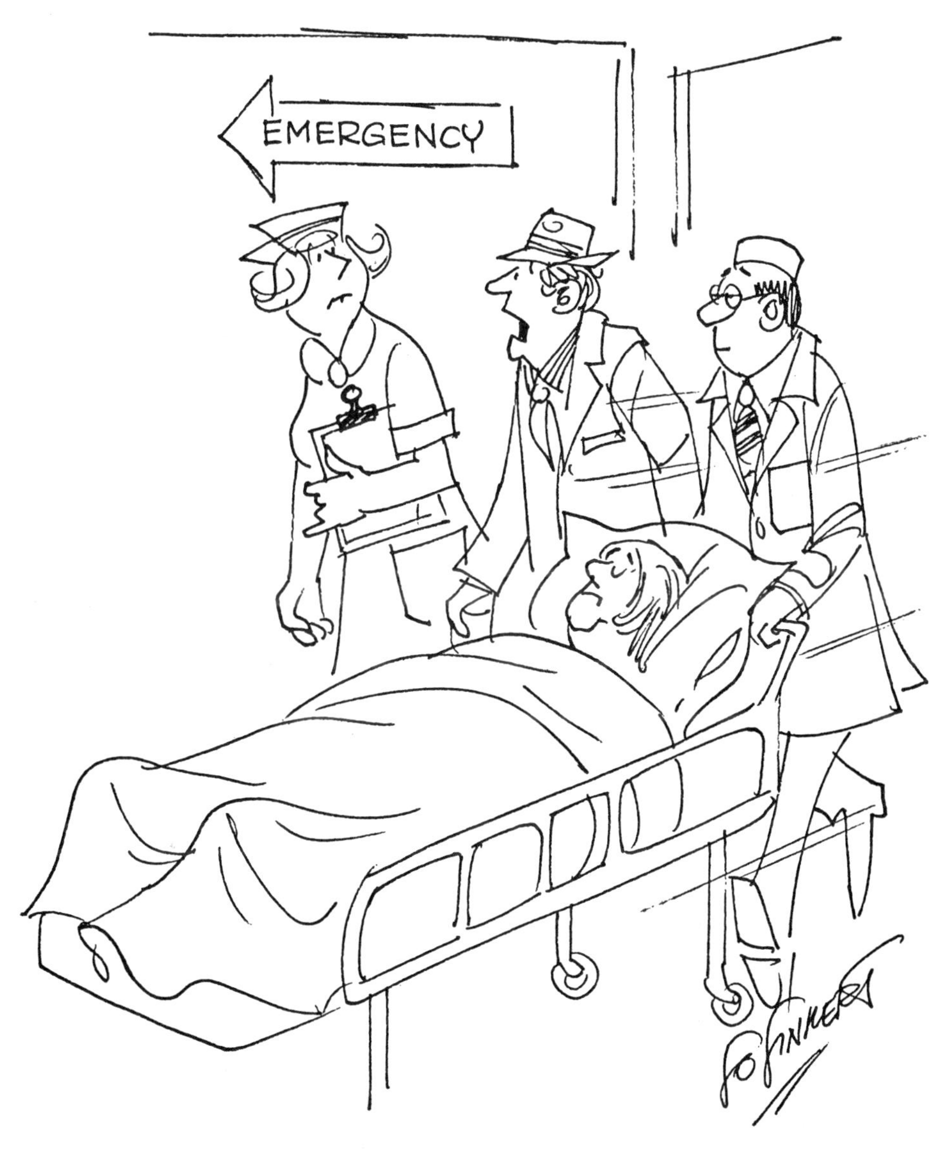

" SHE CRASHED ON HER CRASH DIET."

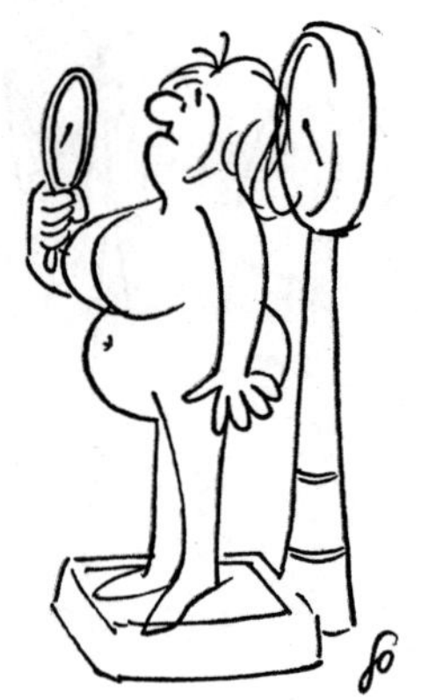

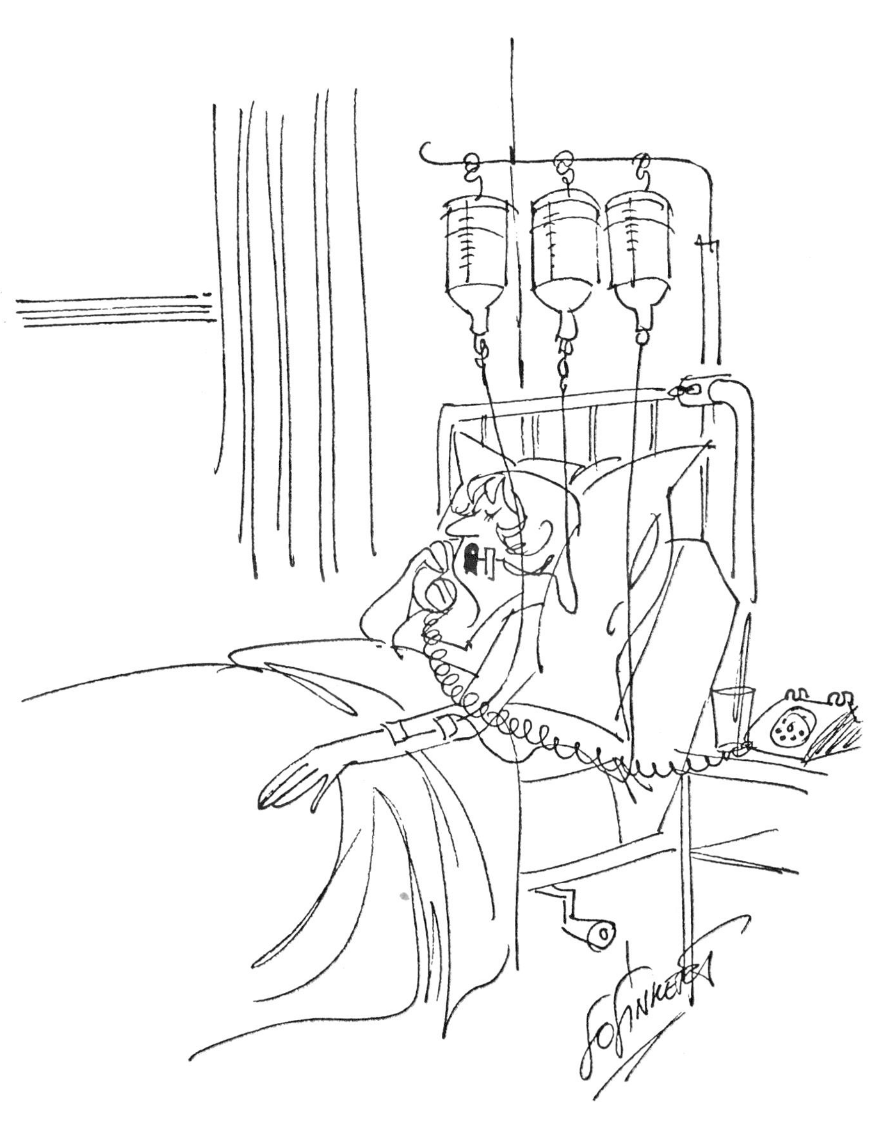

" I'LL CALL YOU BACK WHEN I'M FINISHED EATING."

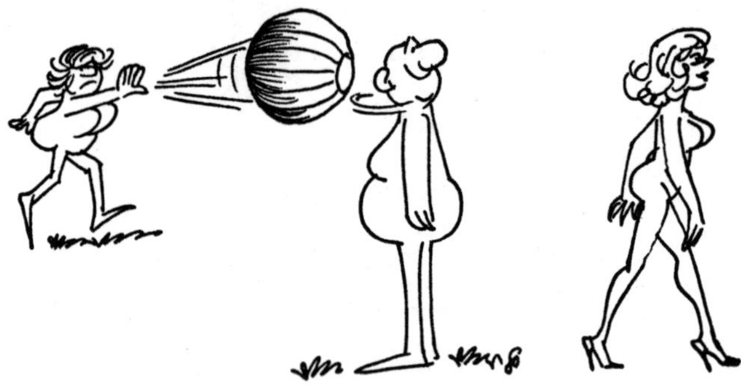

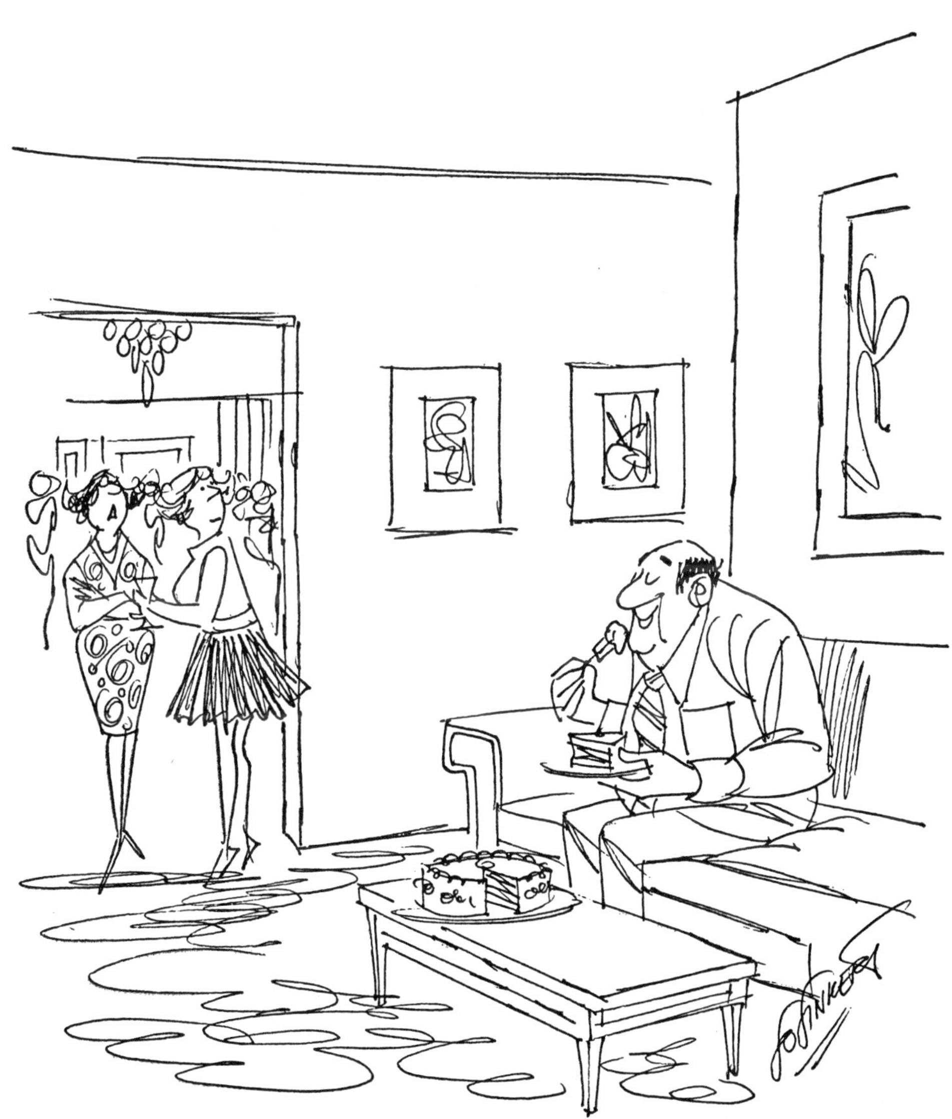

"HOW CAN I PUT HIM ON A DIET WHEN HE GOES AROUND TELLING EVERYONE HOW MUCH HE LOVES TO BE A LIVING TESTIMONIAL TO MY CULINARY ARTISTRY."

MY FAVORITE PEOPLE
ARE THOSE WHO GO ON
A DIET QUIETLY.

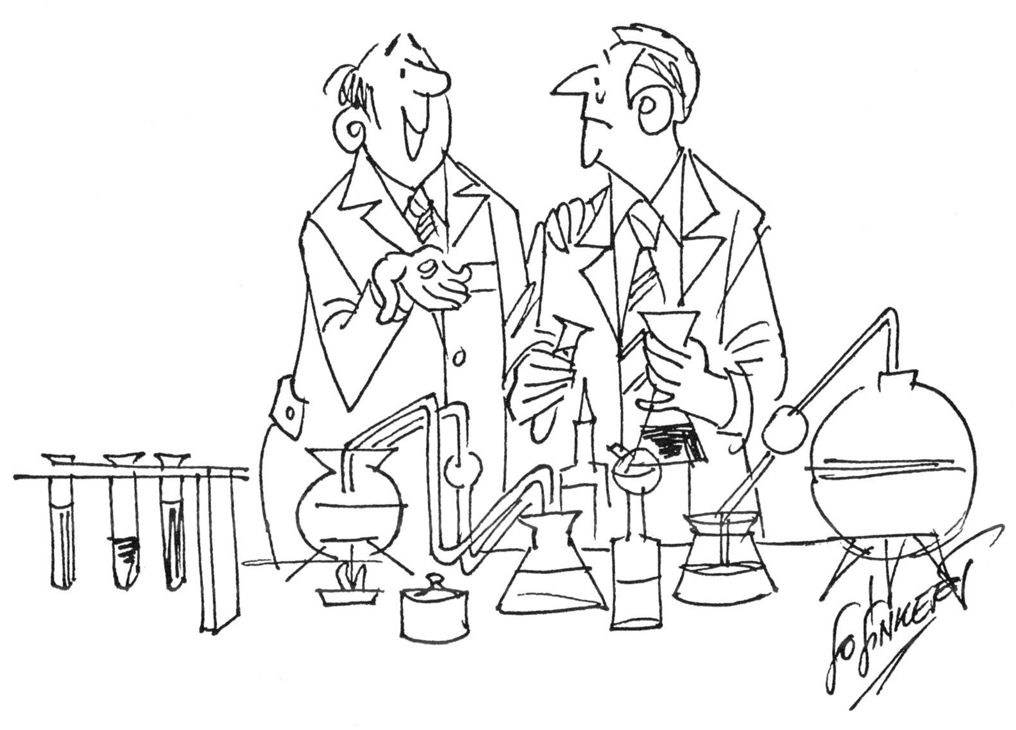

" AT LAST... A SAFE DIET PILL. WHEN YOU FIND OUT HOW MUCH IT COSTS, YOU LOSE YOUR APPETITE."

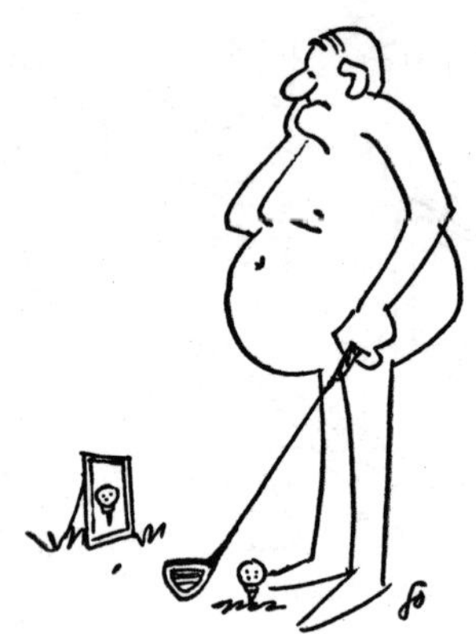

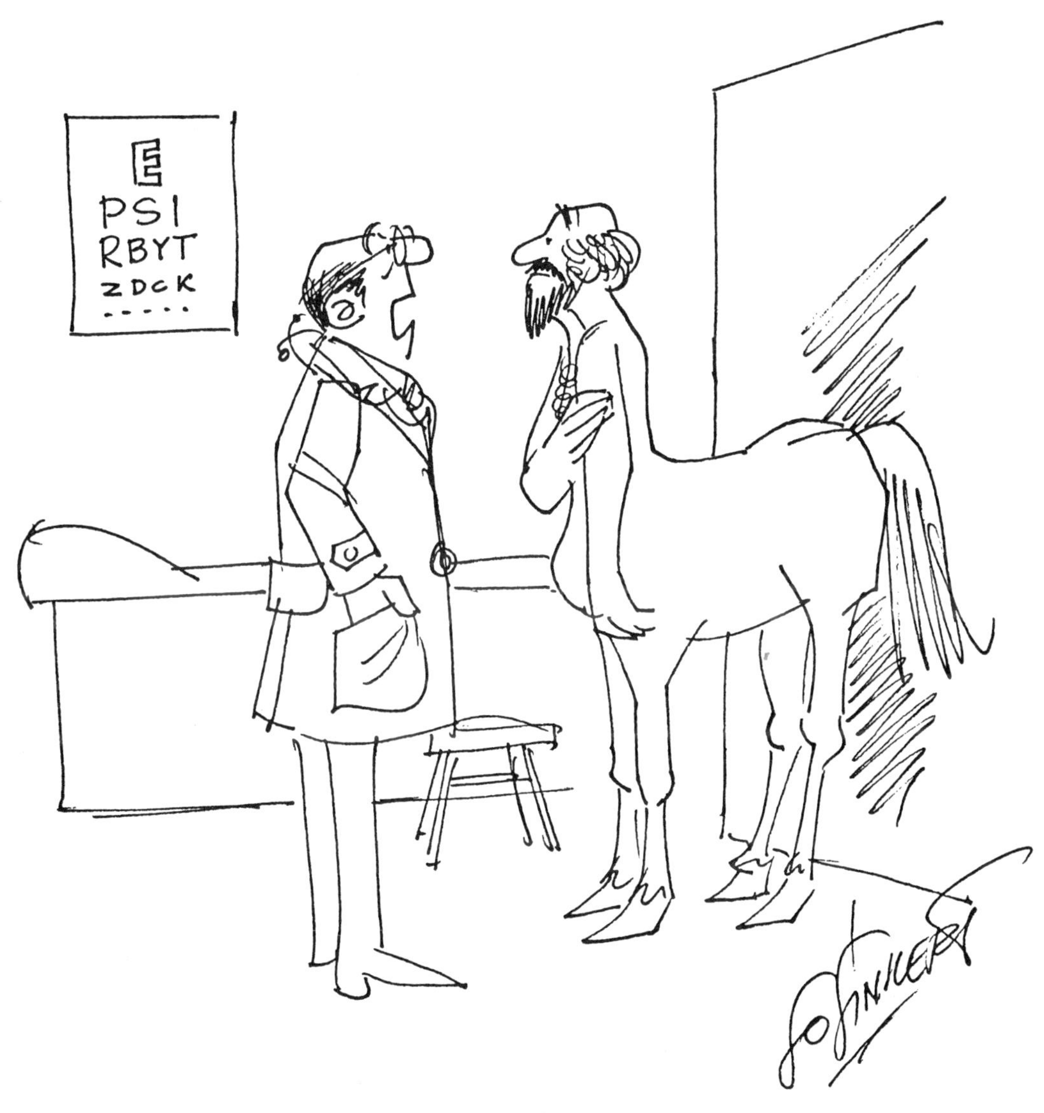

" YOU GOT TO STOP EATING LIKE A HORSE."

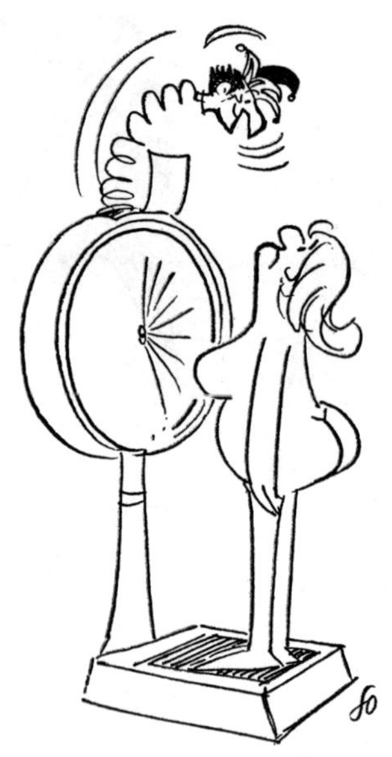

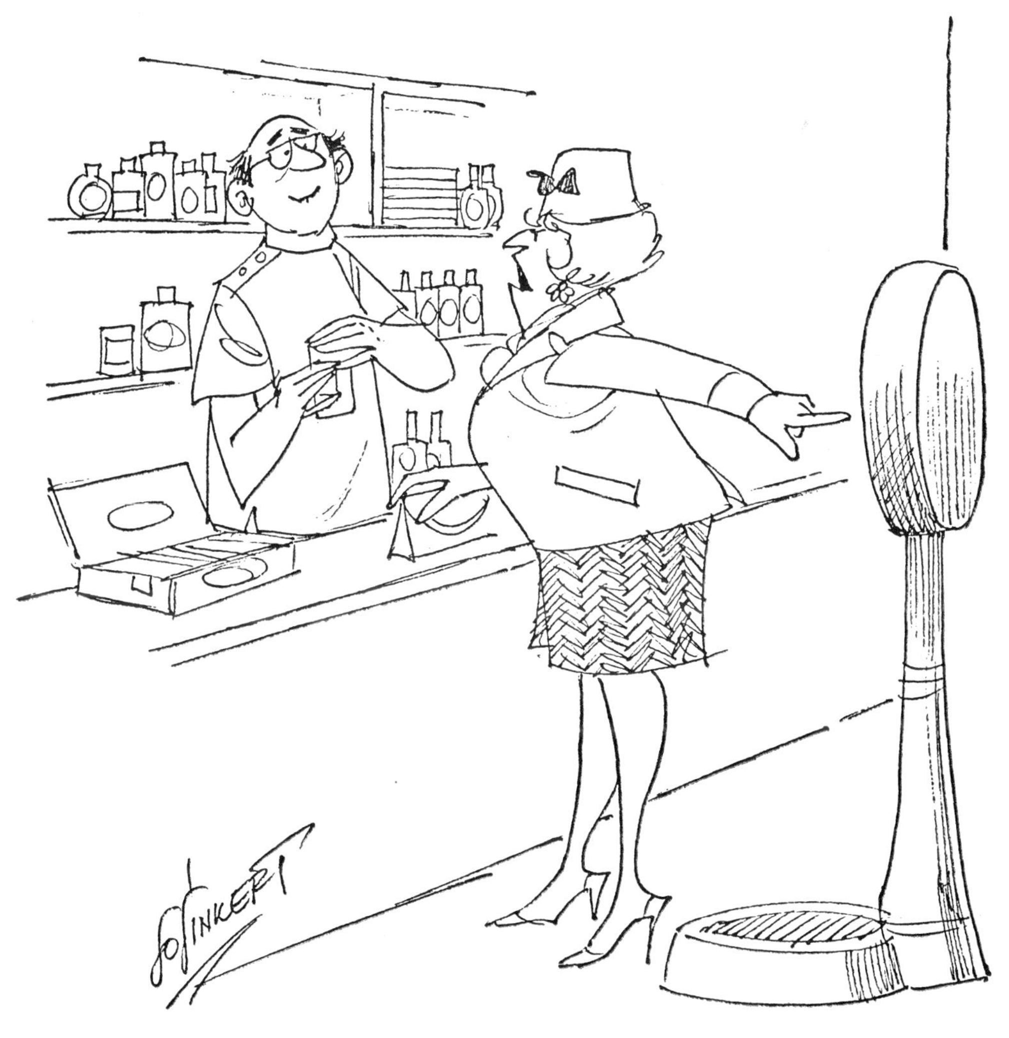

"IT'S SUPPOSED TO GIVE ME A CARD WITH MY WEIGHT AND FORTUNE ON IT, BUT ALL I GOT WAS CANNED LAUGHTER!"

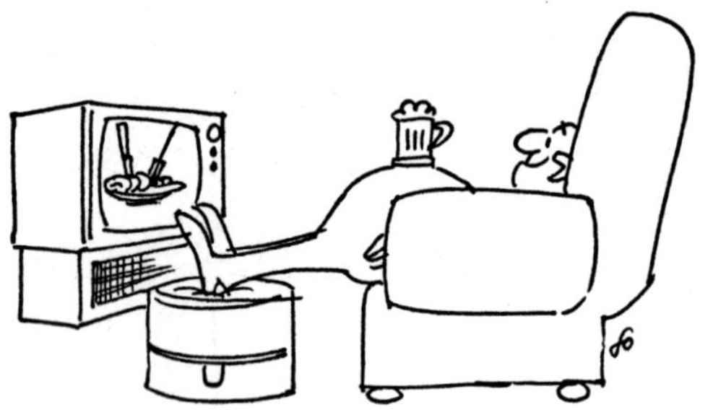

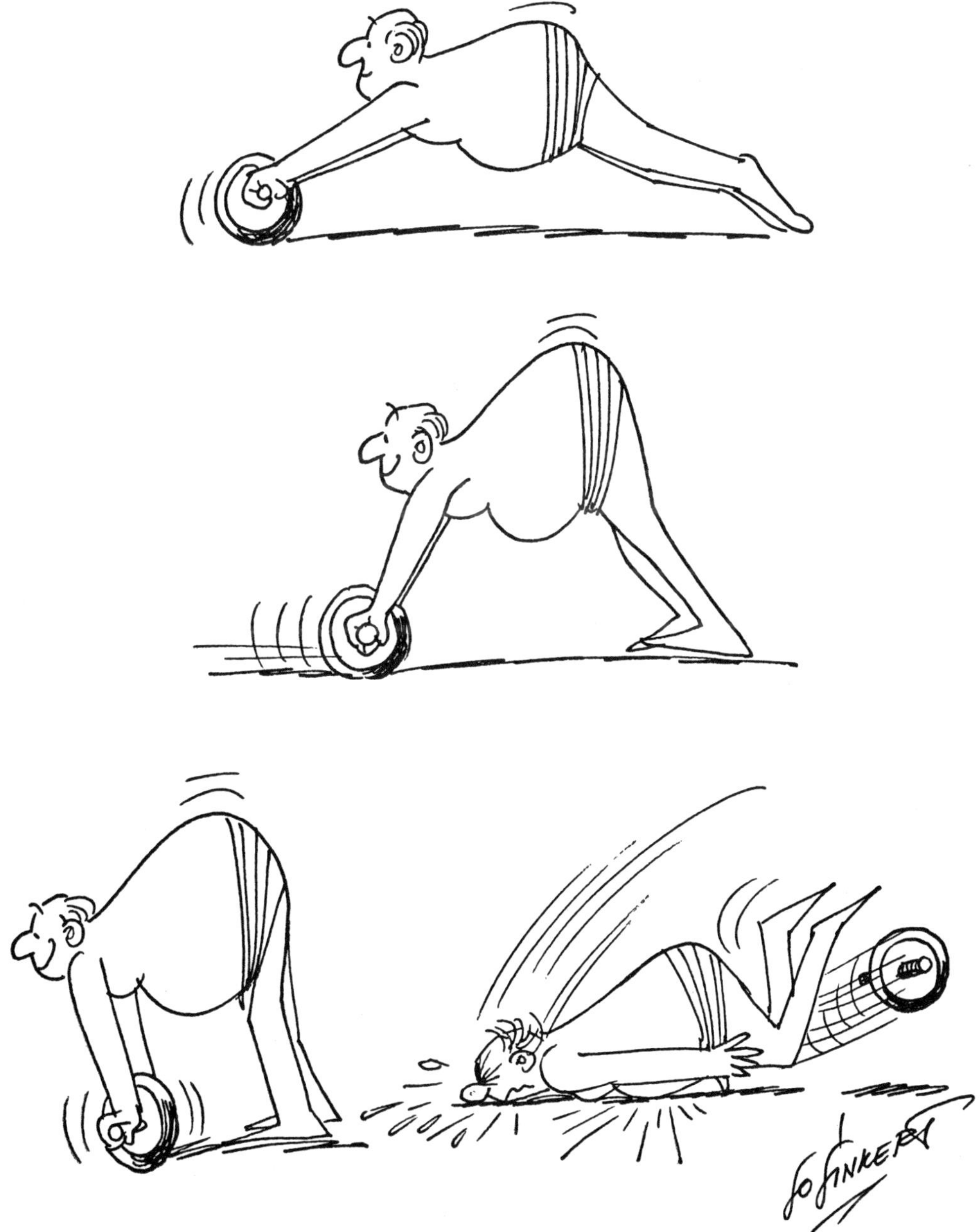

A SURE WAY TO LOSE WEIGHT IS TO PUT COTTON IN YOUR EARS - YOU WON'T HEAR THEM YELL 'COME AND GET IT.'

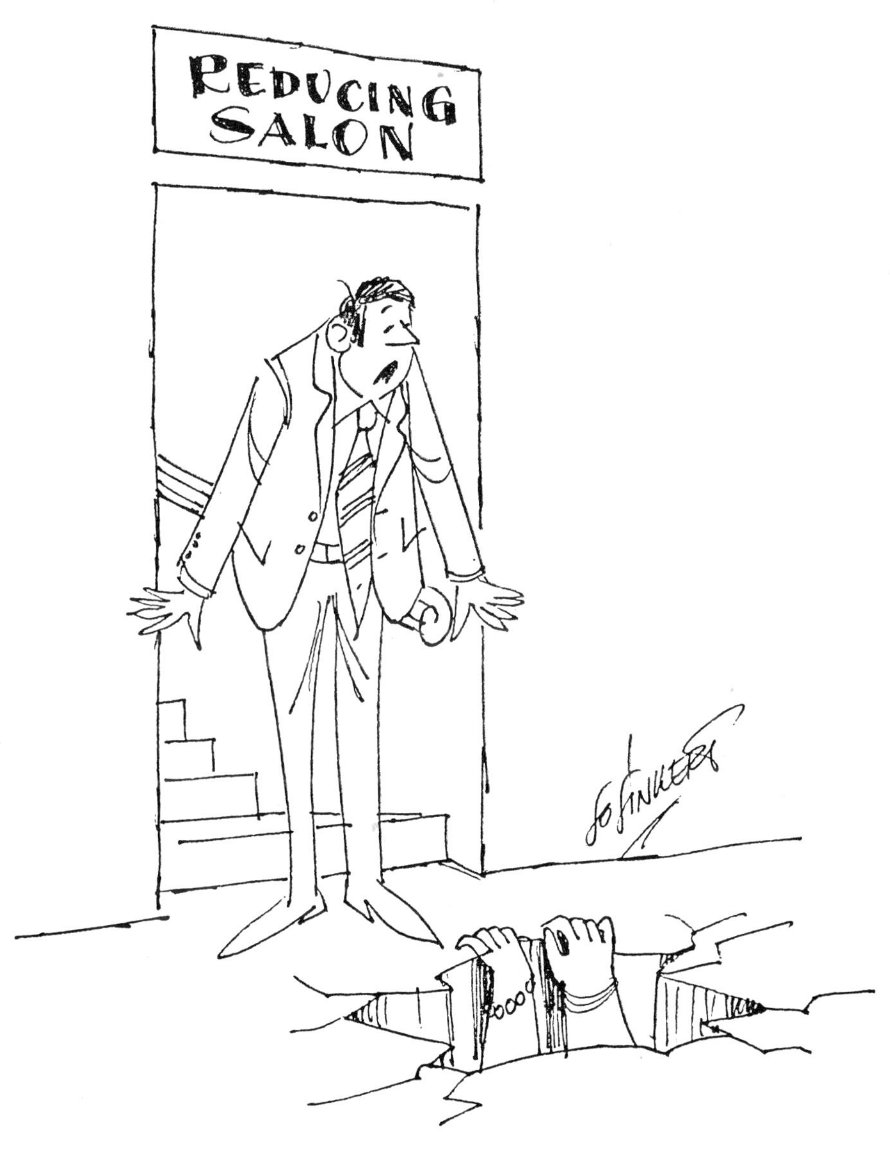

"YOU SHOULD HAVE COME EARLIER MS. DARBY."

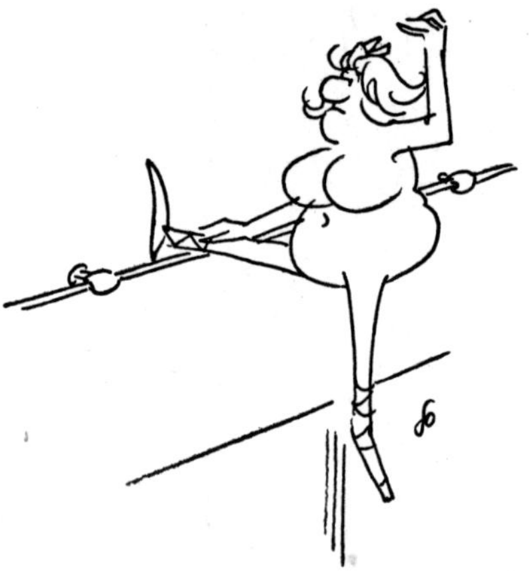

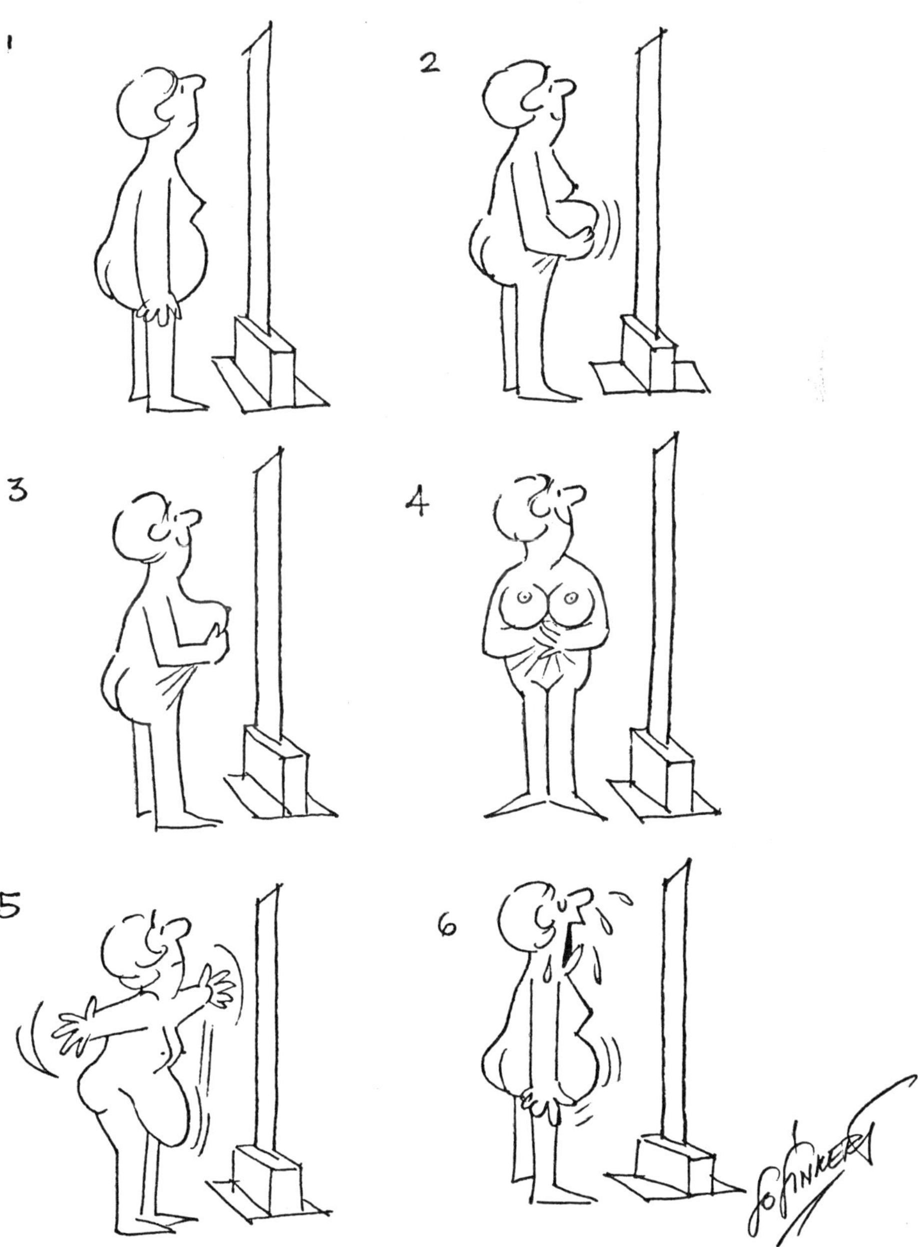
1
2
3
4
5
6

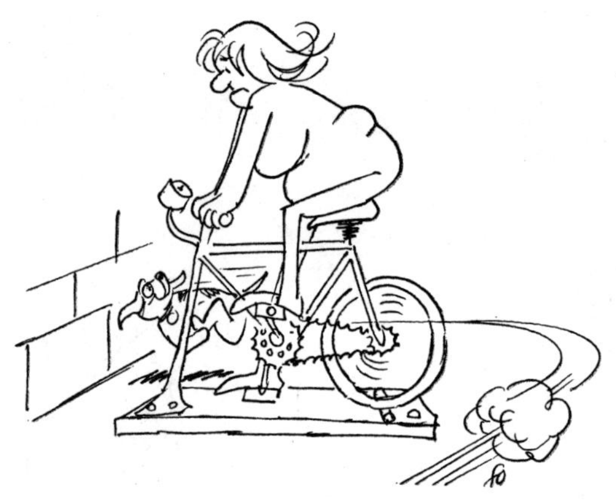

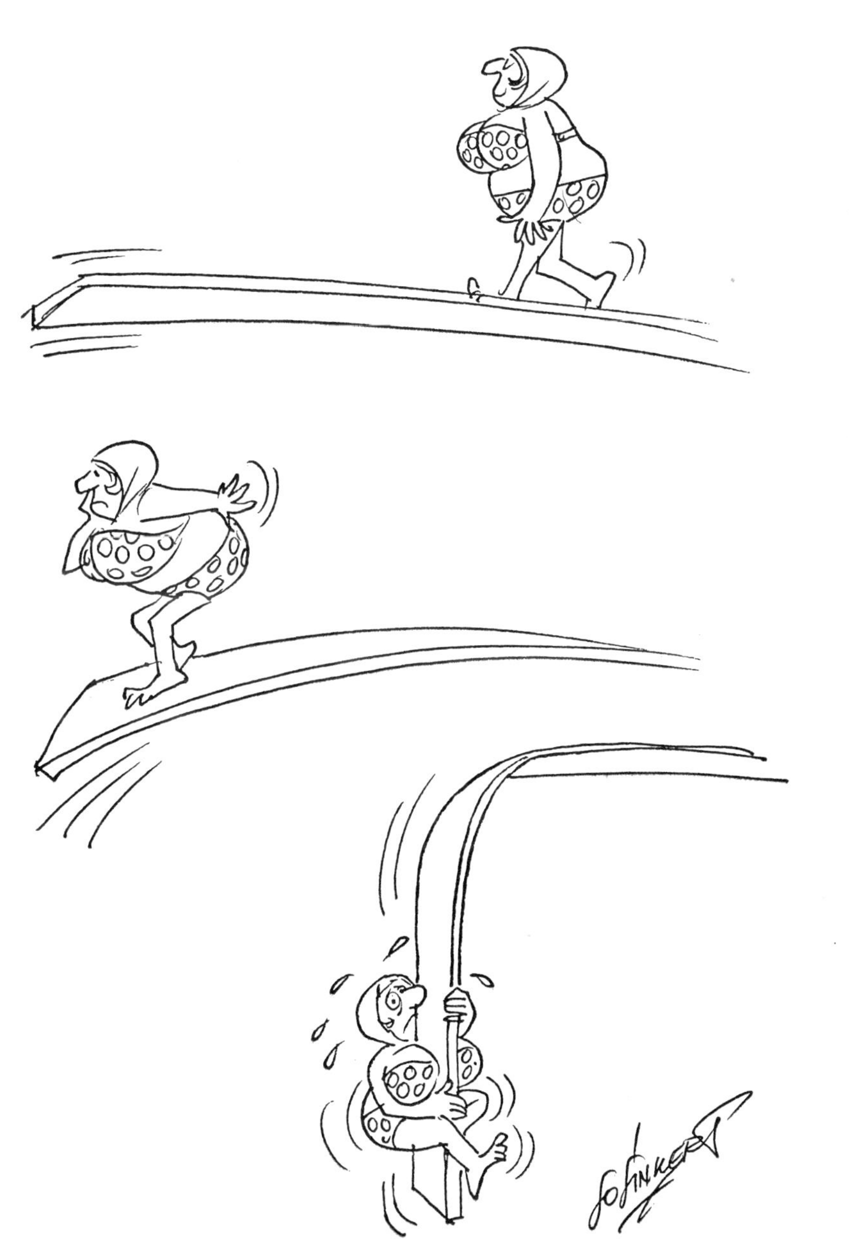

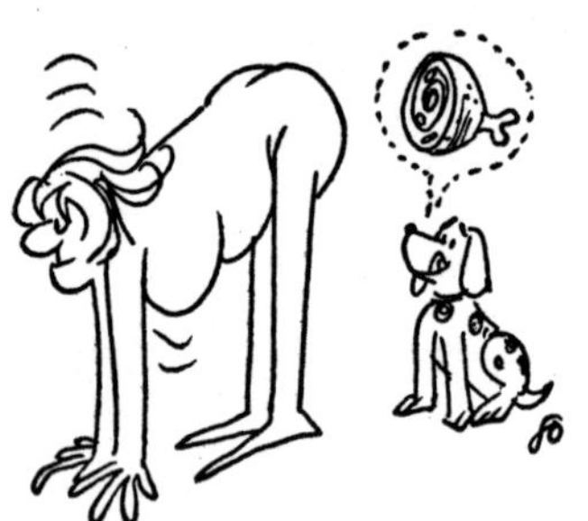

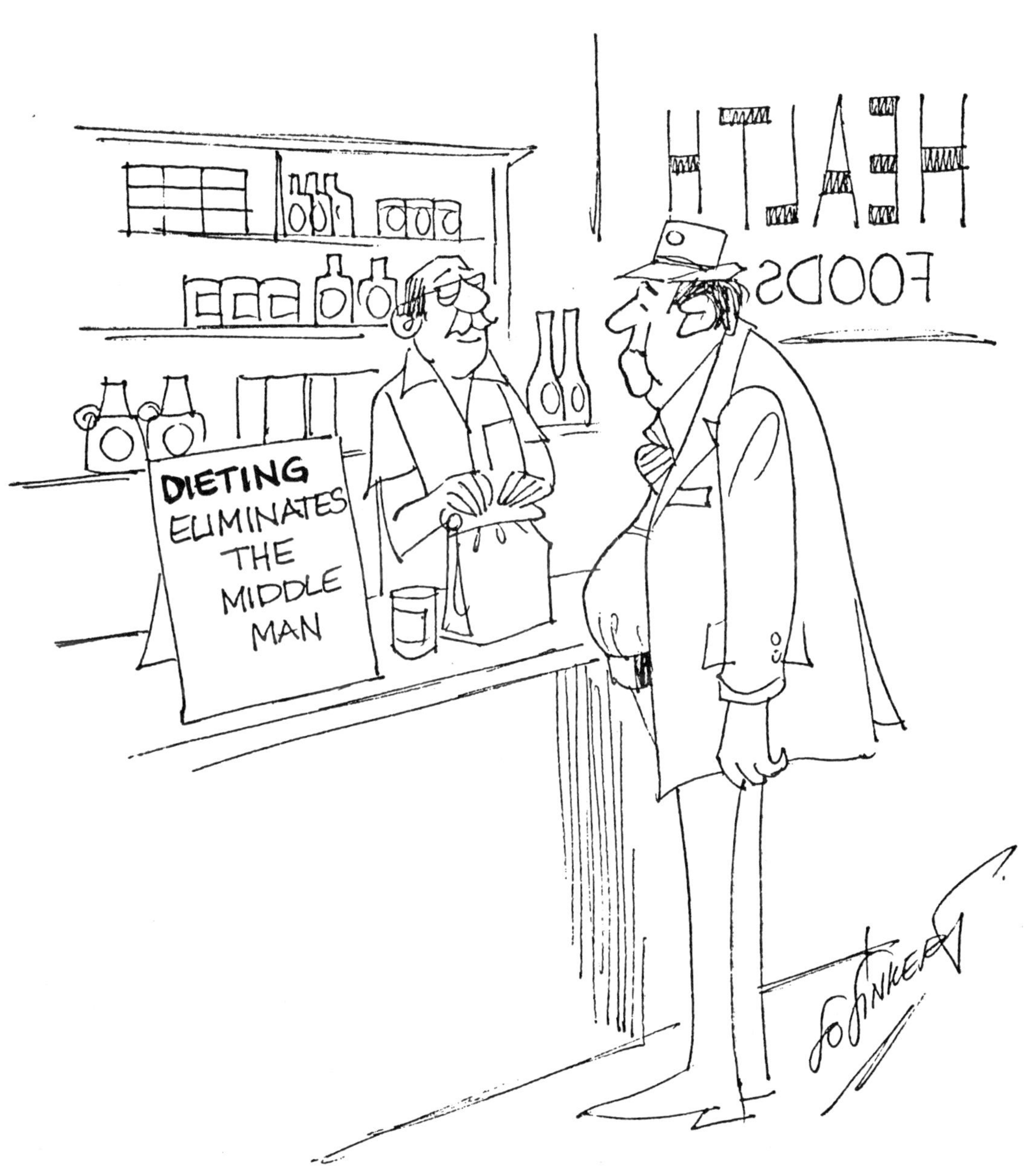
HEALTH
FOODS
DIETING ELIMINATES THE MIDDLE MAN

STRETCHPANTS ARE
STRETCHPANTS BECAUSE
THEY HAVE NO OTHER CHOICE.

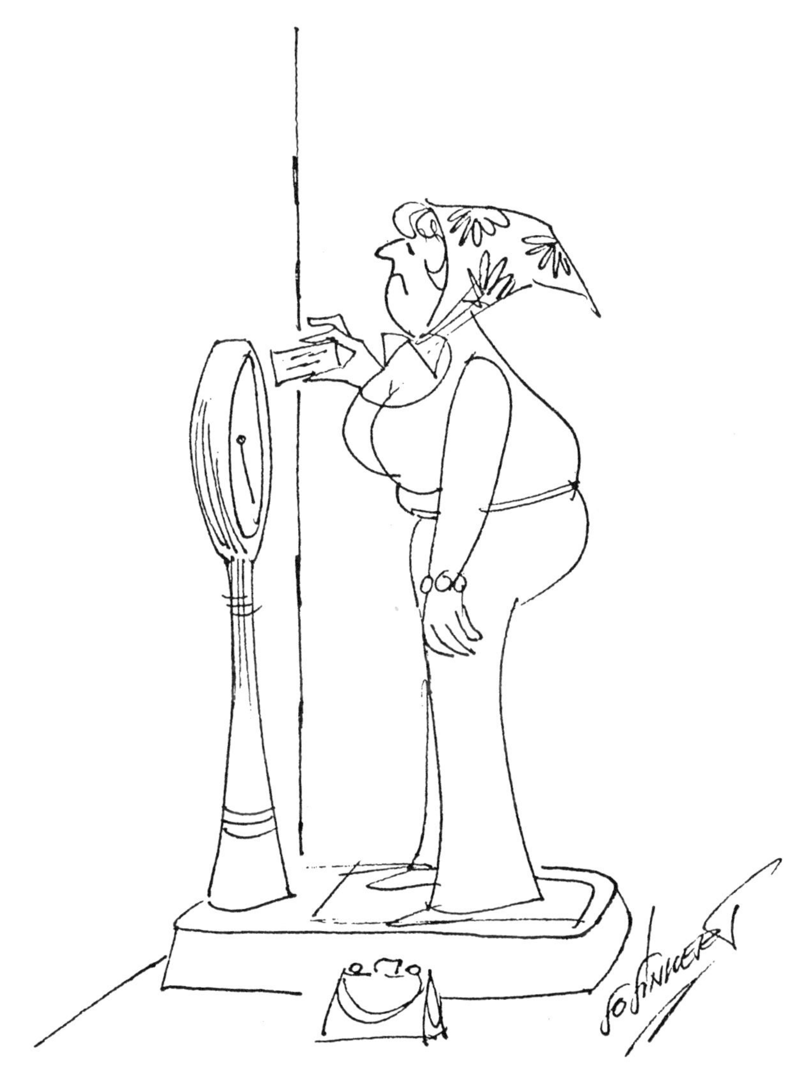

"CARD IS GOOD FOR ONE FREE HALF HOUR GLORIA'S REDUCING SALON."

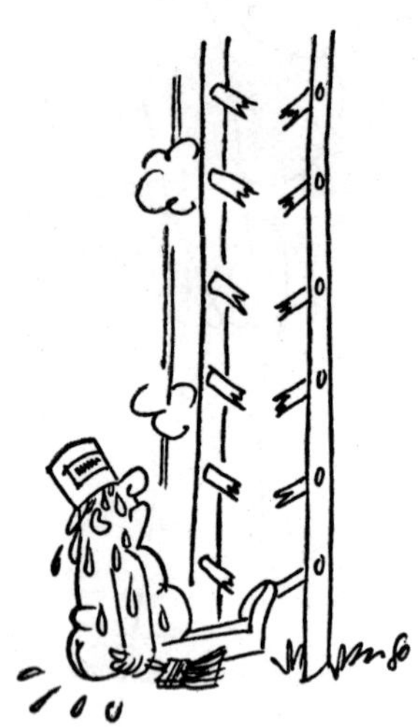

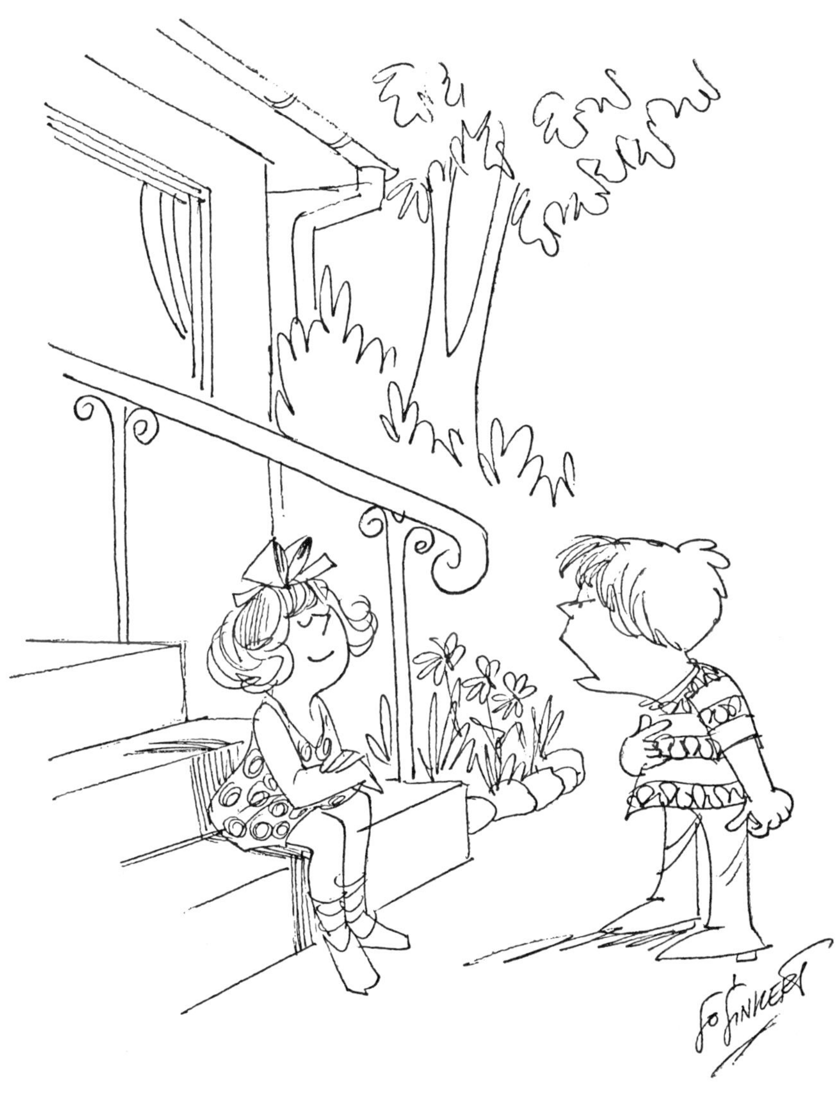

" OH YEAH? MY DAD COULD OUT-JOG YOUR MOM ANY DAY."

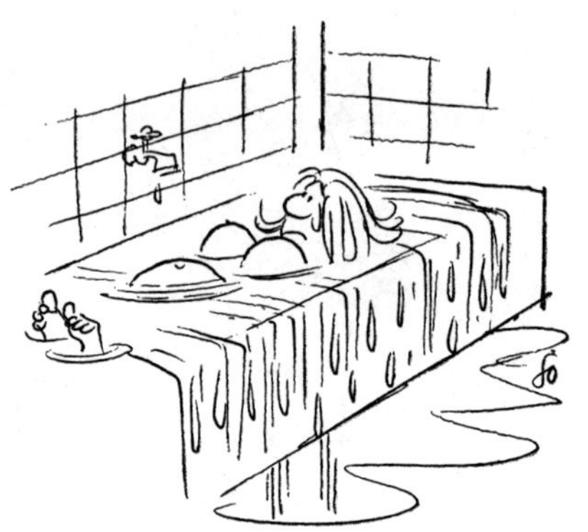

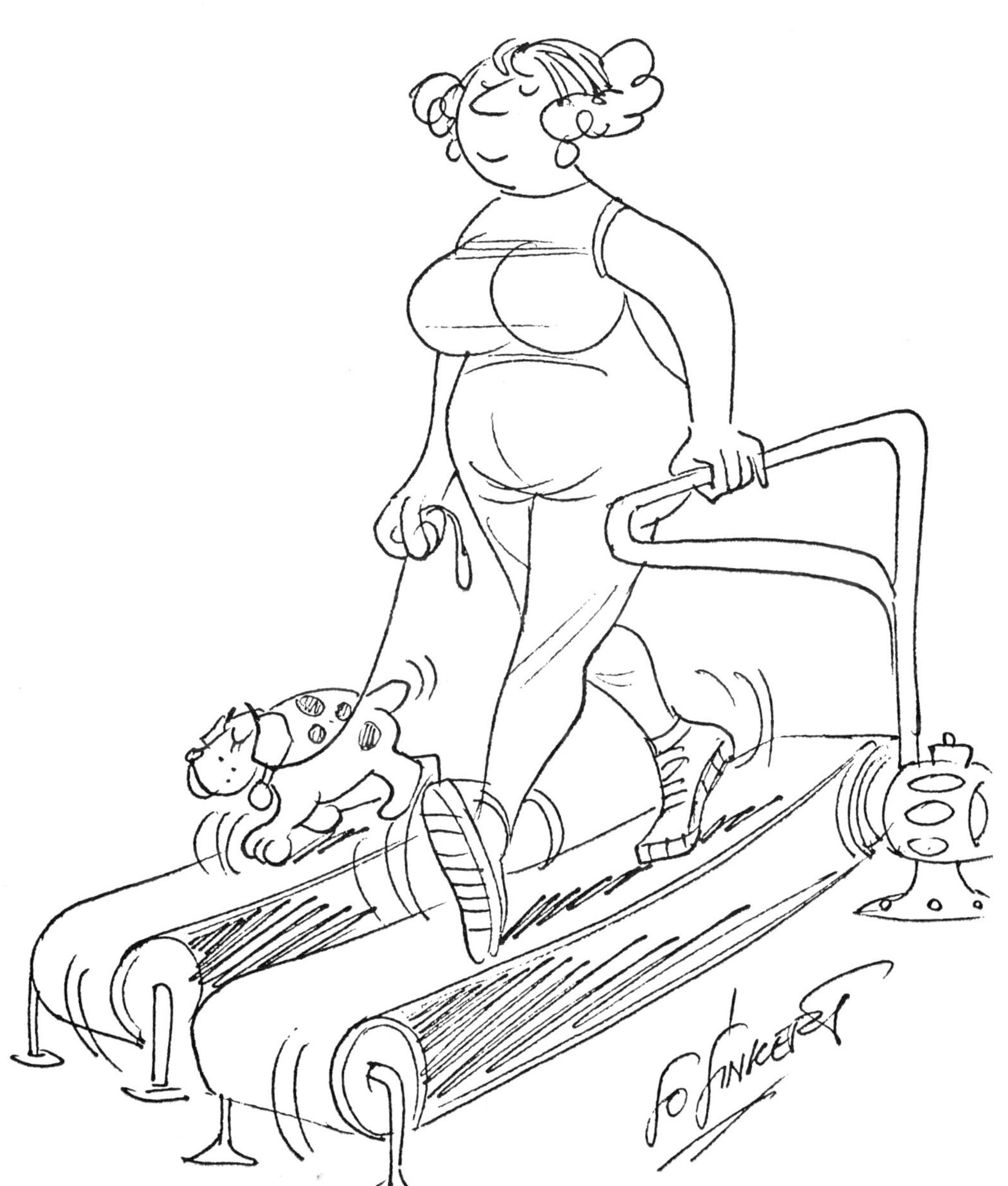

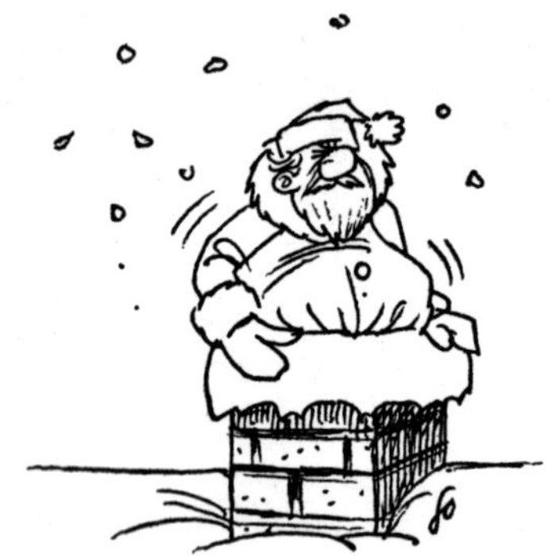

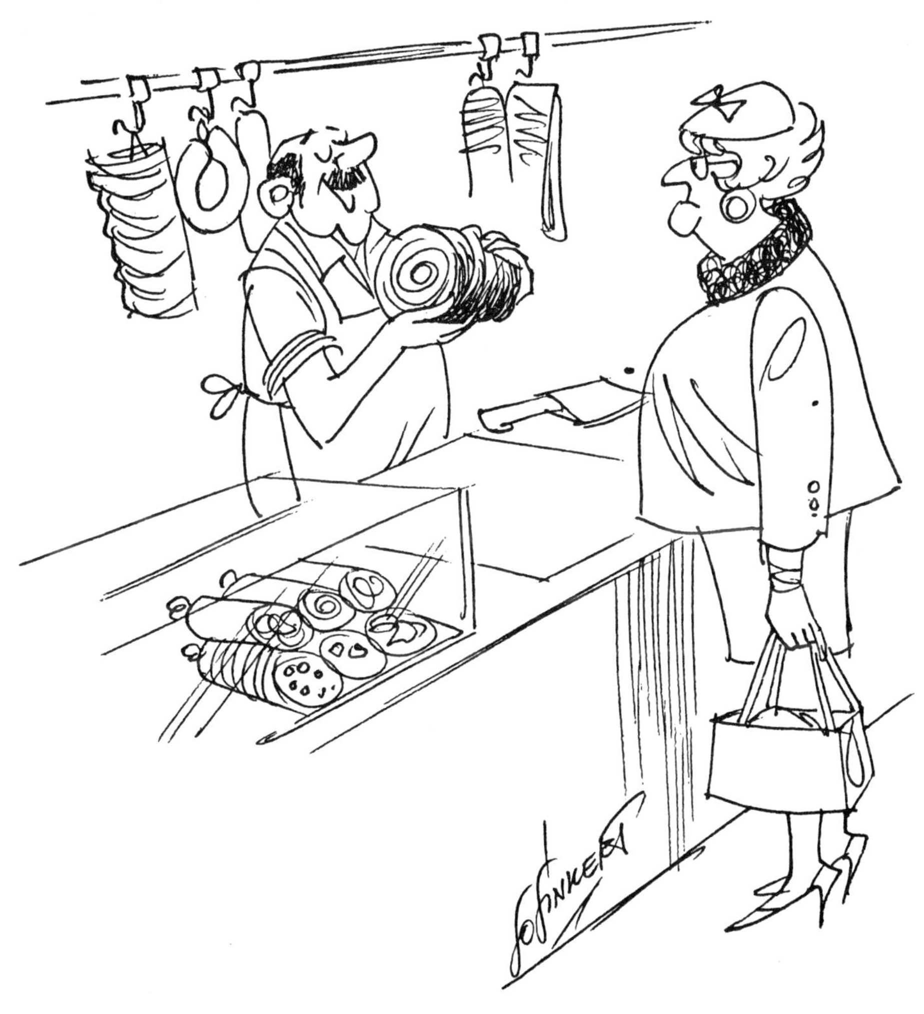

"BELIEVE ME, MRS. ROSSBOROUGH, YOU'LL NEVER SEE A FINER RUMP UNLESS YOU STAND IN FRONT OF A THREE-WAY MIRROR."

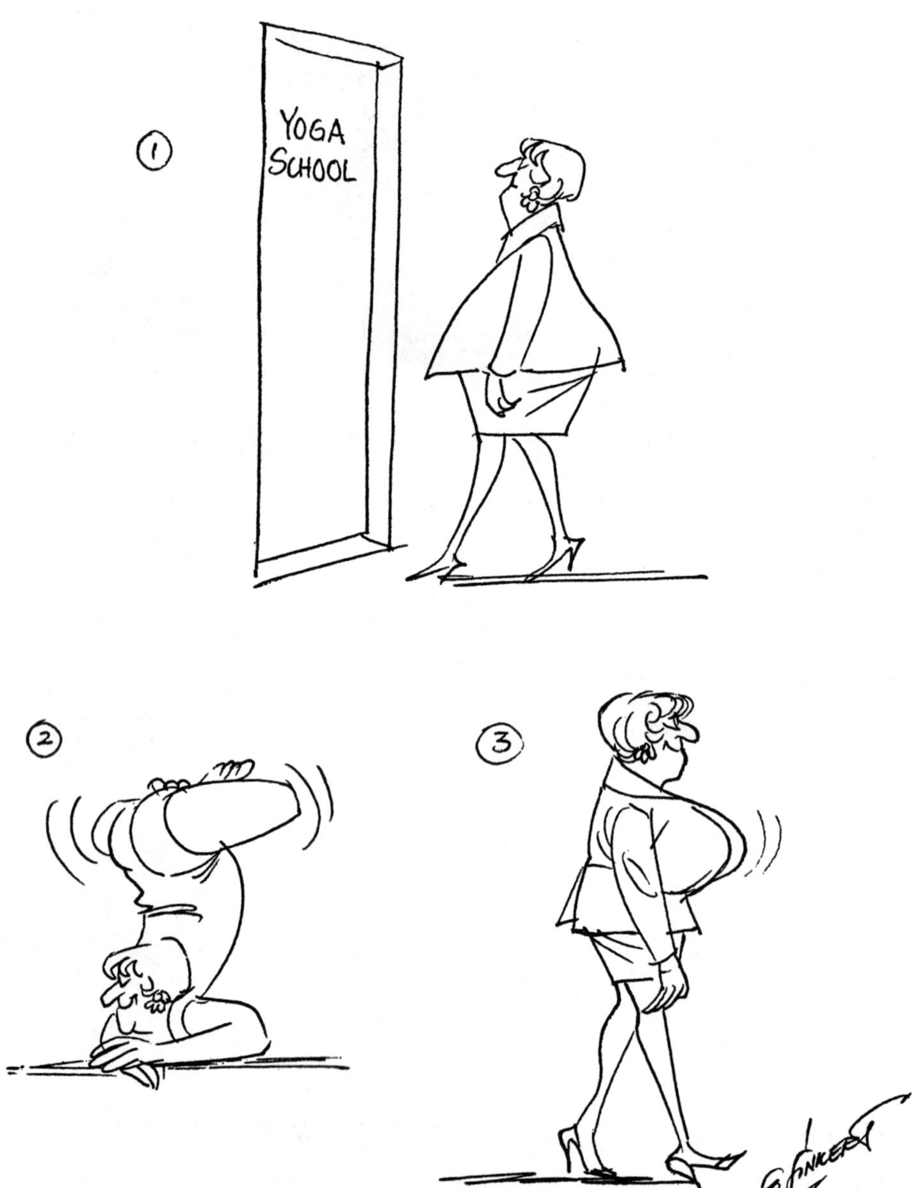
1
YOGA SCHOOL
2
3
JO PINKERT

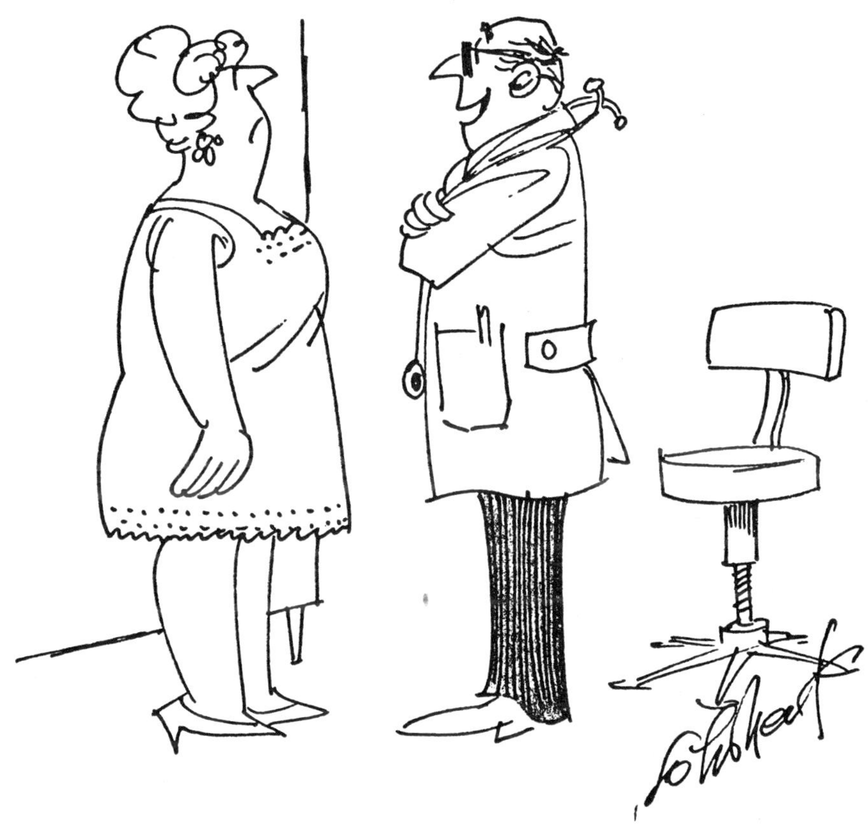

" THE 'THREE SQUARES' A DAY I WAS REFERRING TO ARE CRACKERS."

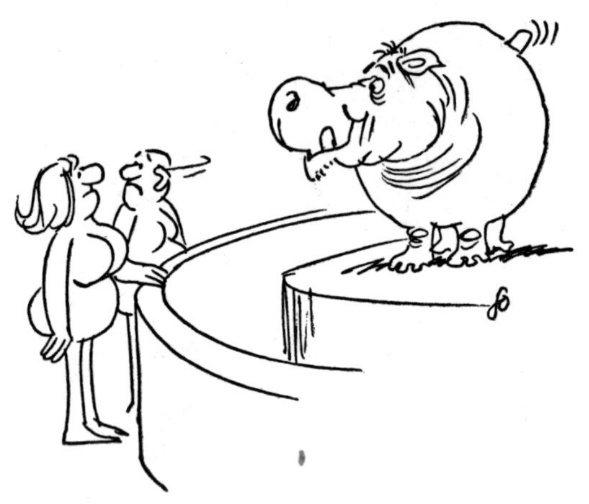

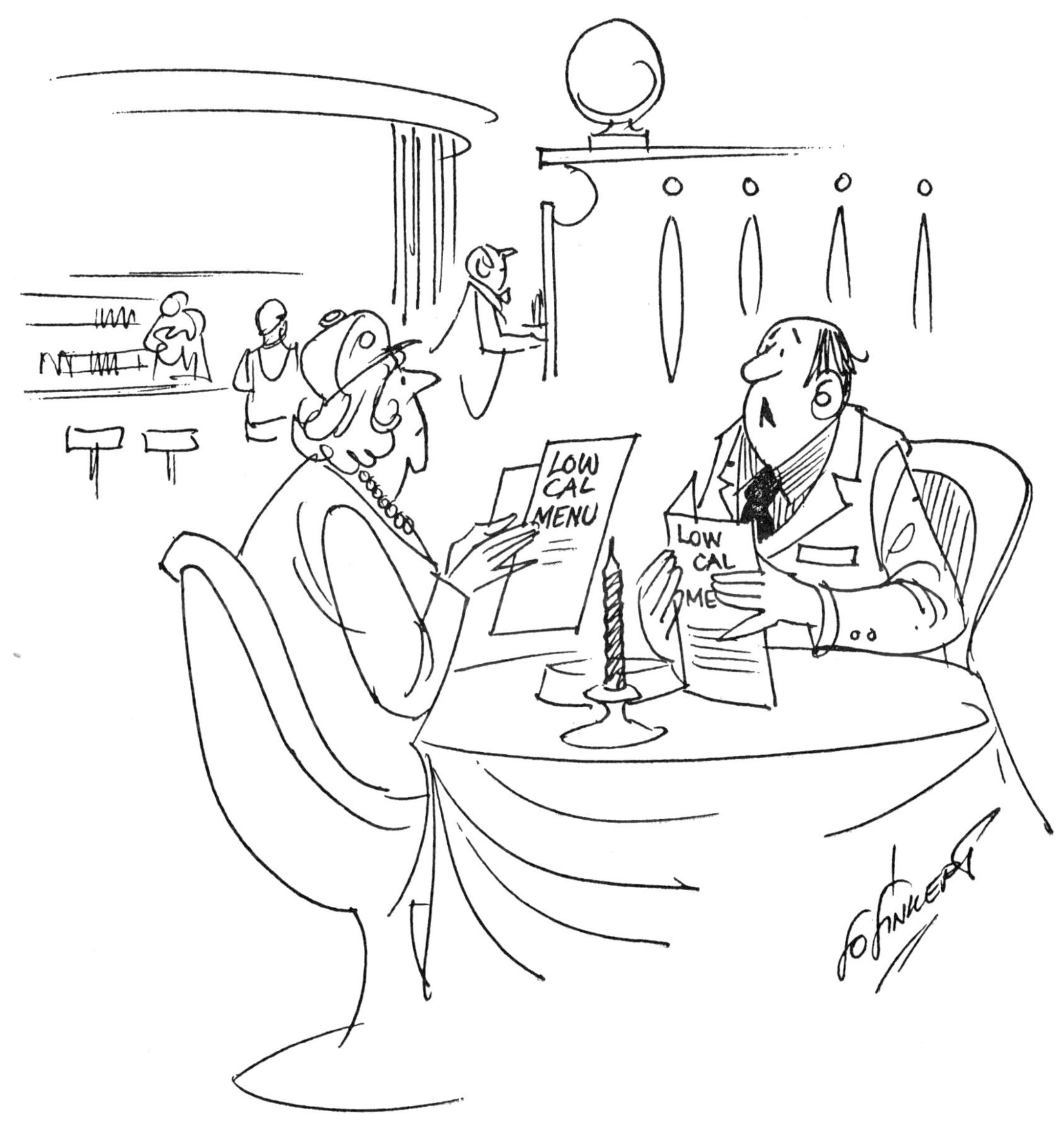

"CLAIRE, DO YOU REALIZE THAT IS 10¢ A CALORIE?"

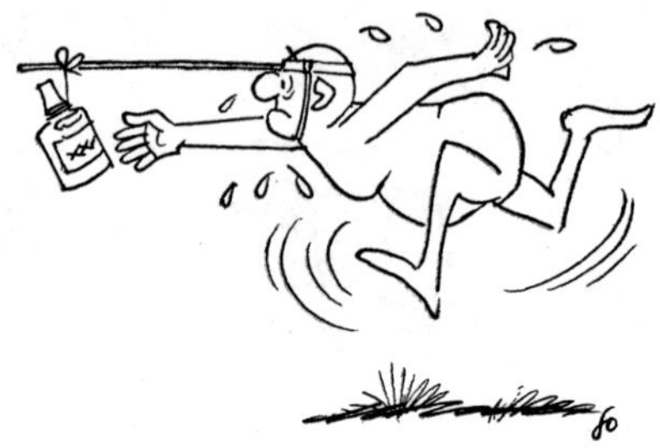

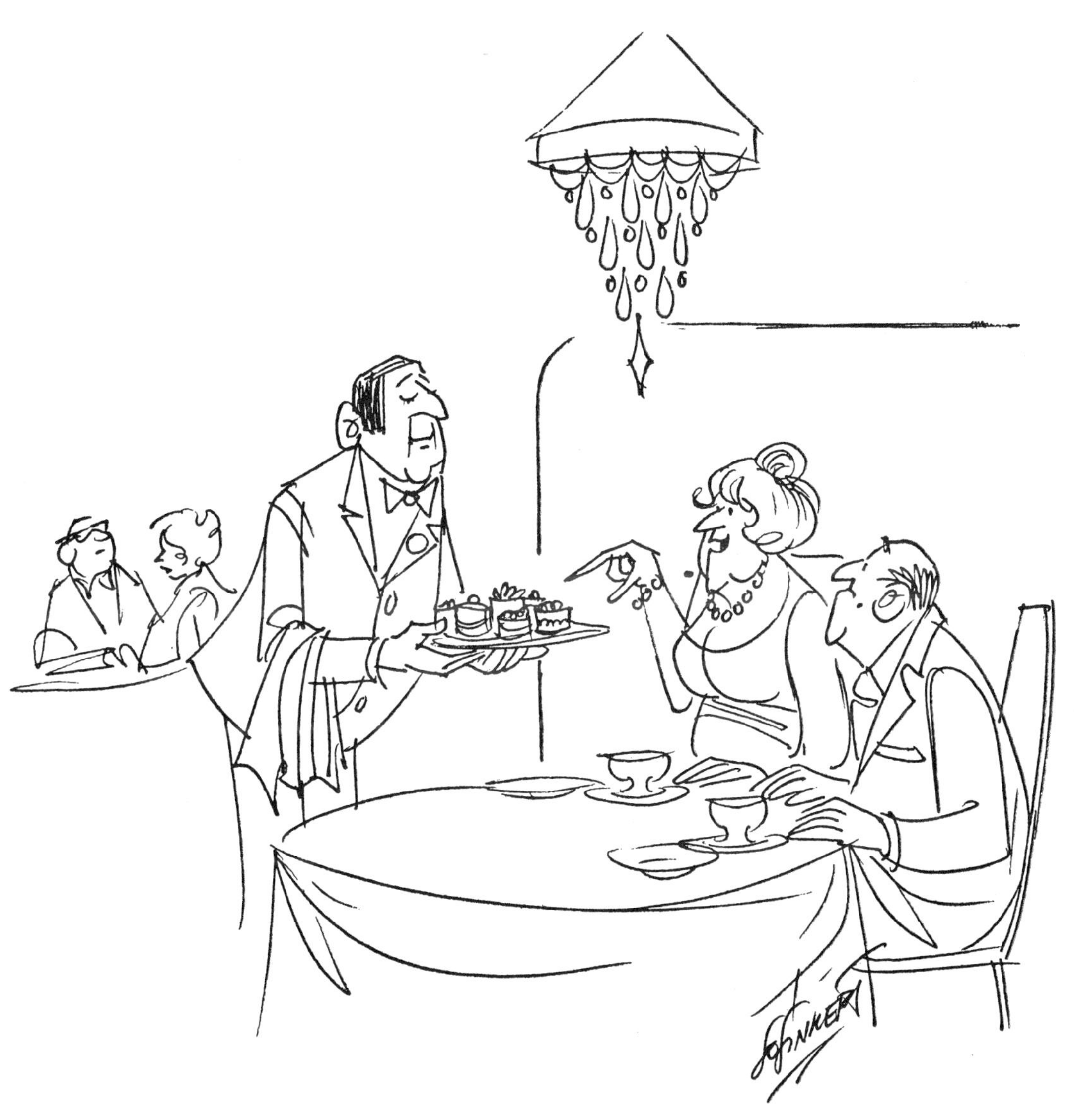

" EENIE, MENIE, MINIE, MO, I'LL TAKE THOSE FOUR. "

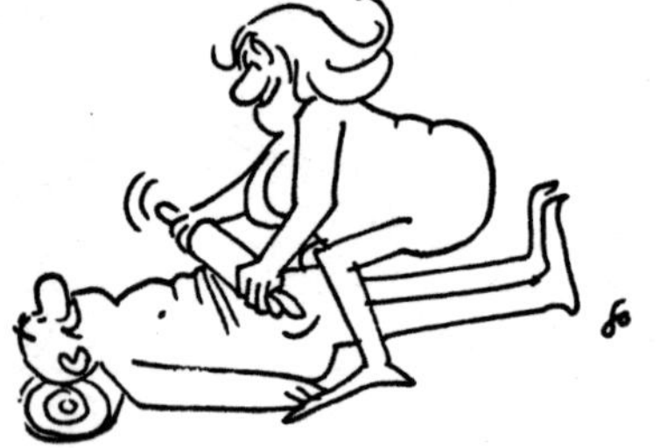

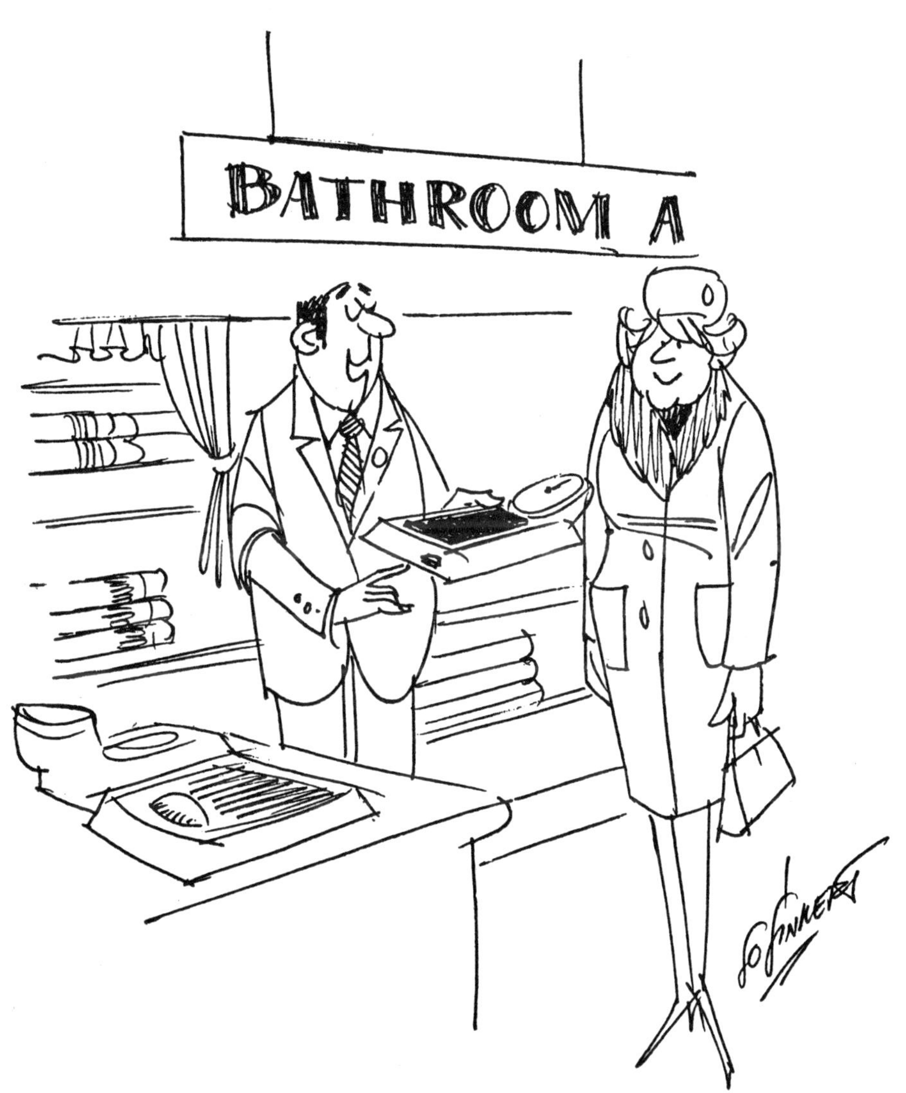

"... THEN FOR YOUR HUSBAND'S USE, YOU JUST KICK THIS LITTLE KNOB."

THE TROUBLE WITH
HEALTH SPAS IS THAT
THEIR HIGH MEMBERSHIP
FEES MAKE YOU SICK.

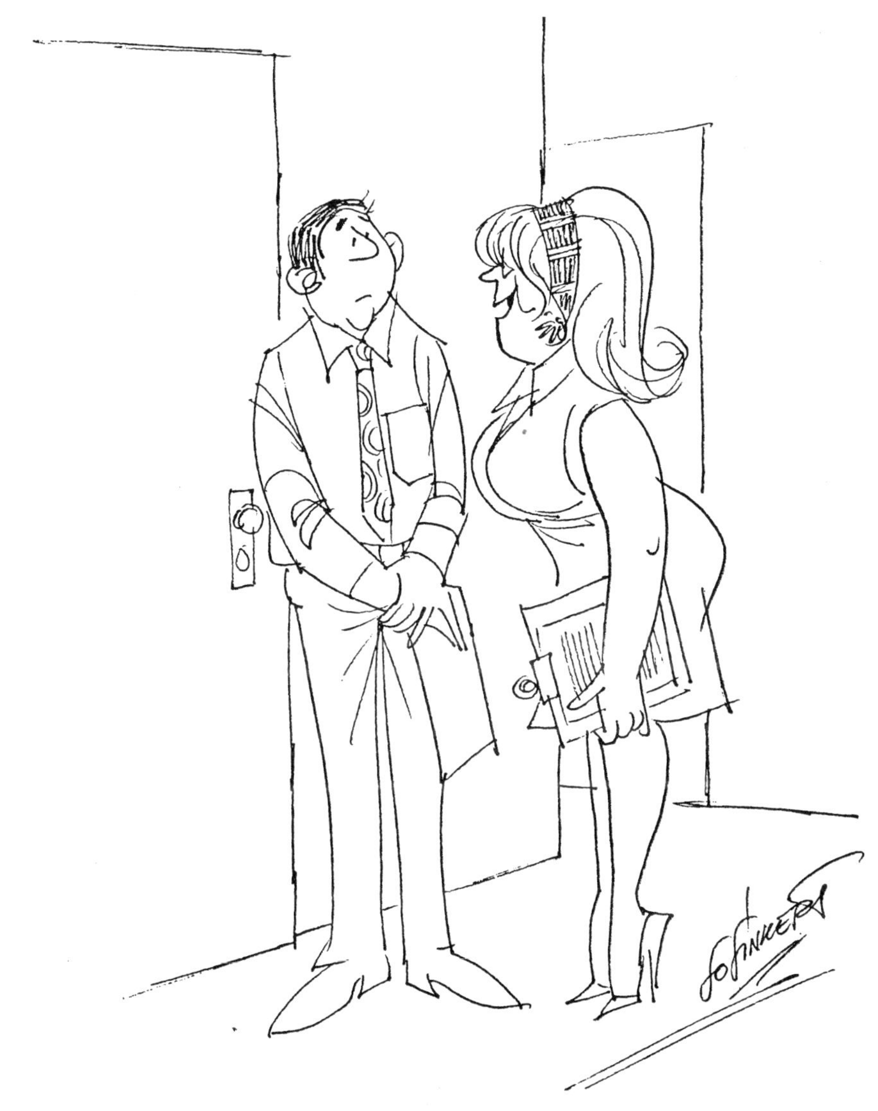

" OF COURSE I HAVEN'T LOST ANY WEIGHT. I'M ON THE NEW 'WHAT-THE-HECK-ENJOY-YOURSELF' DIET."

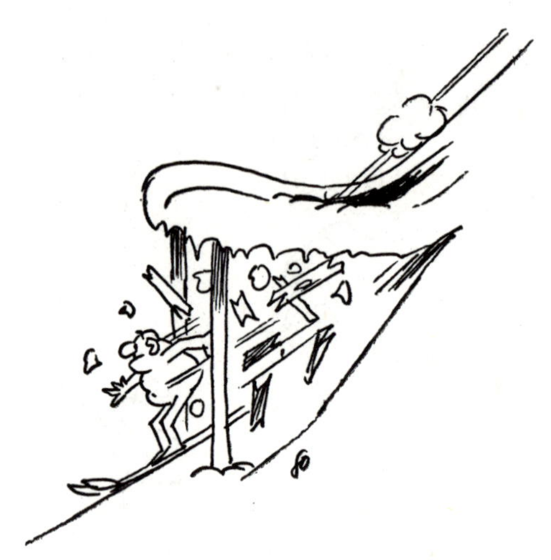

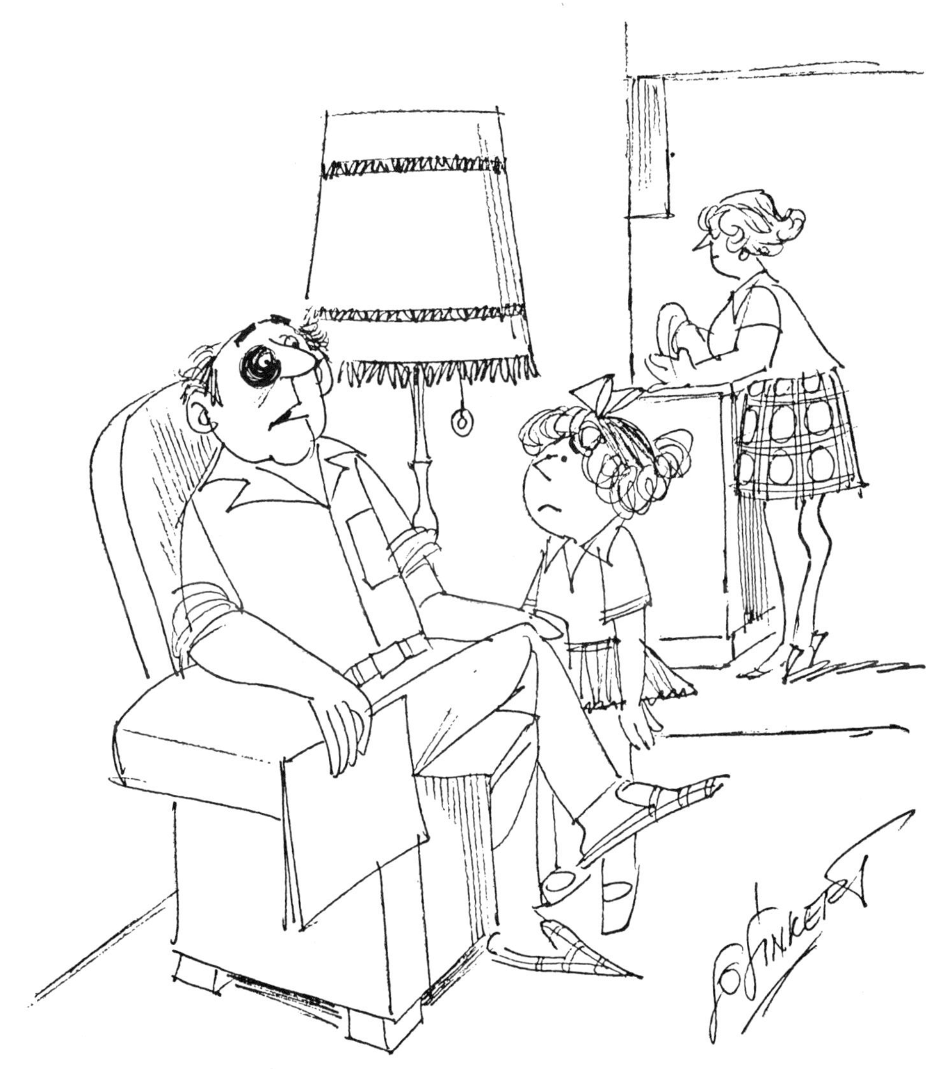

"NEVER MIND WHERE I GOT IT – BUT LET ME WARN YOU – DON'T EVER ASK YOUR MOM HOW MUCH SHE WEIGHS."

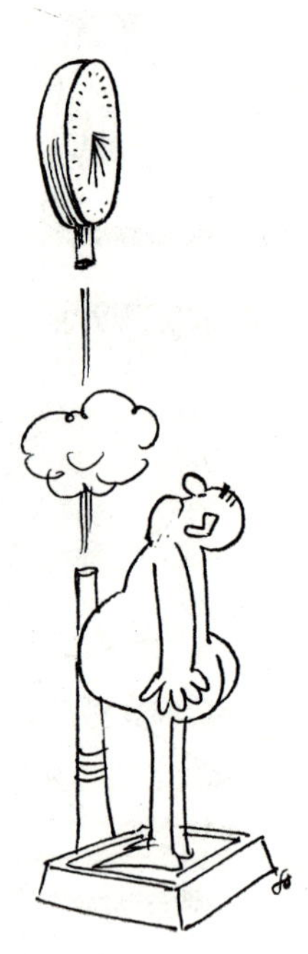

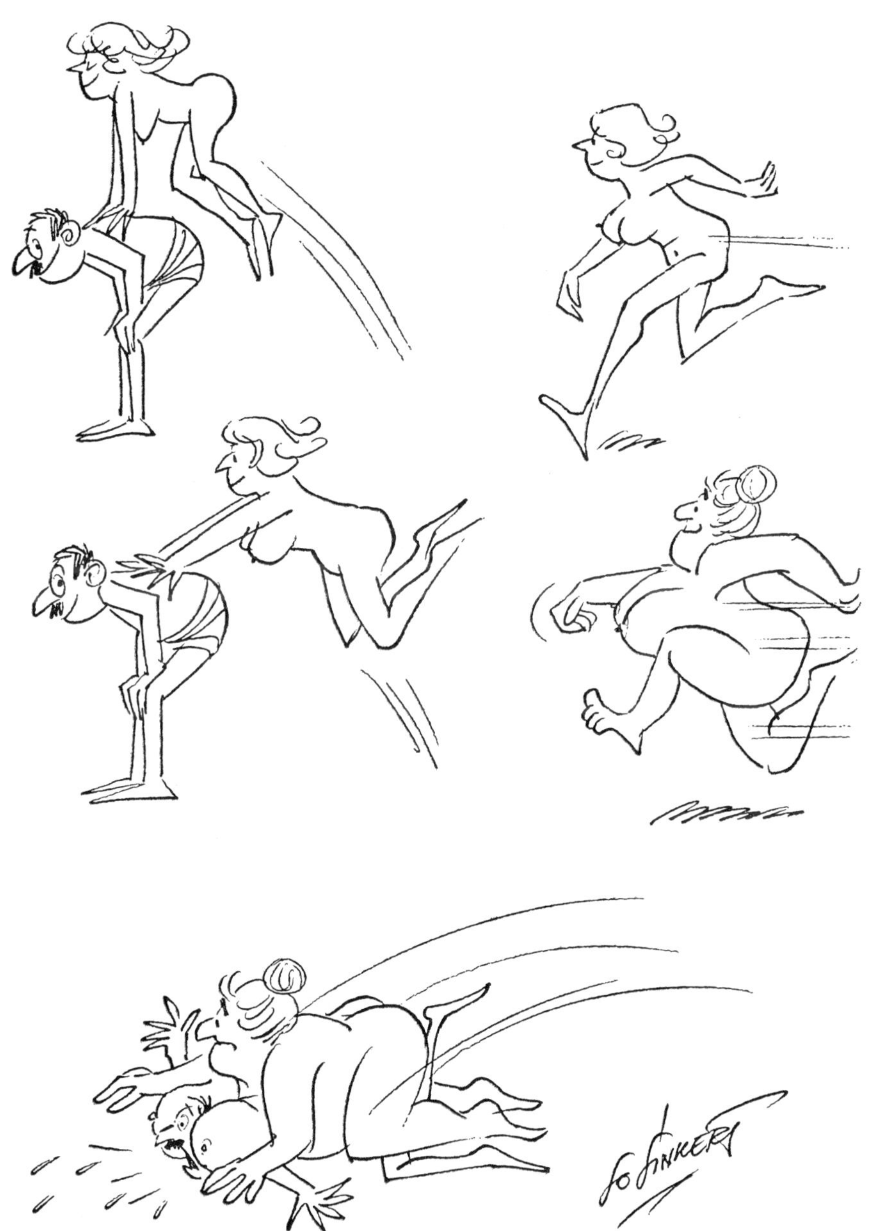

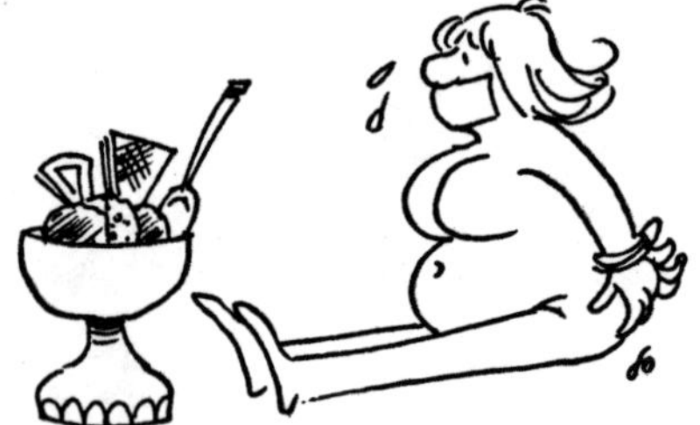

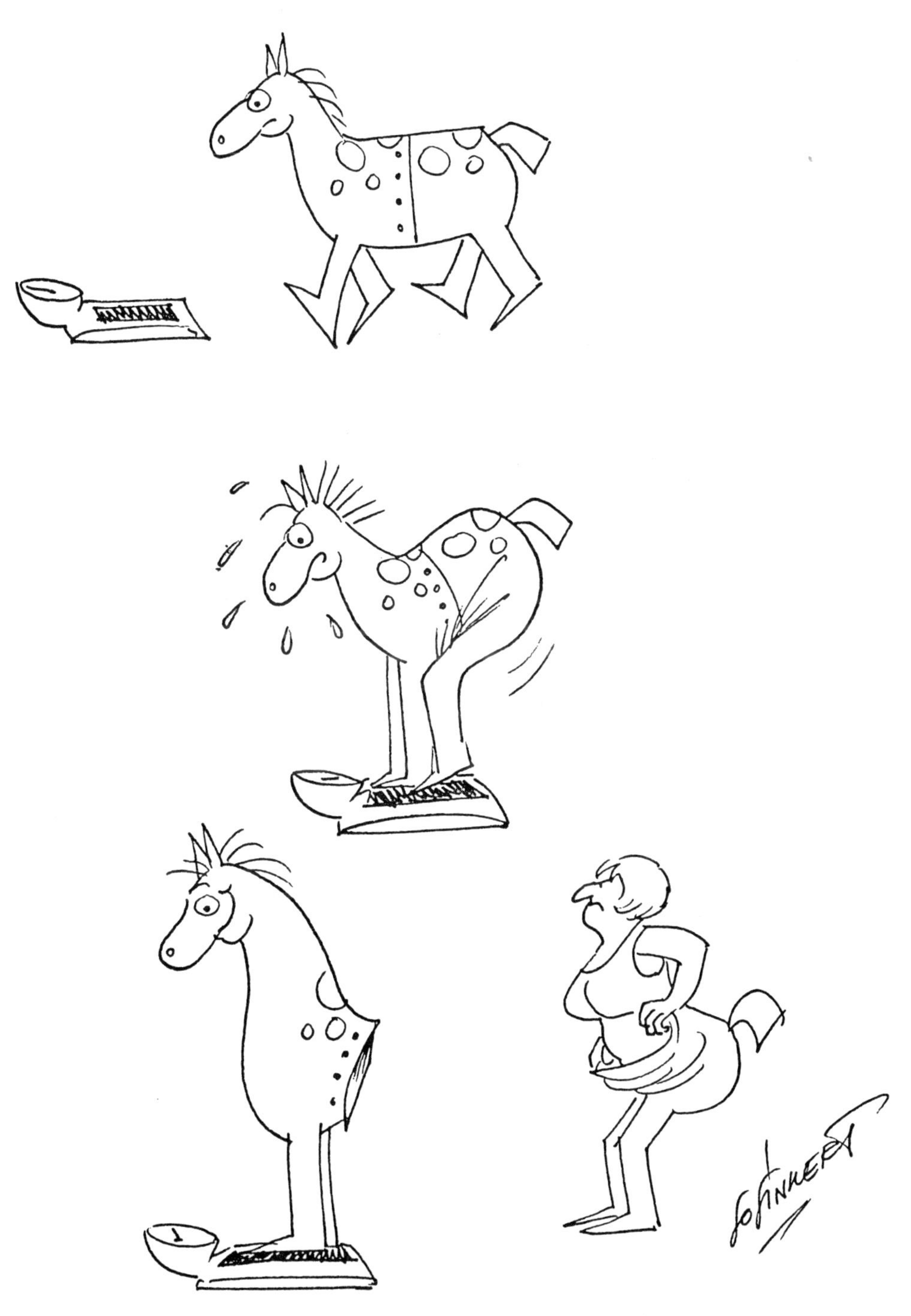

FAT PEOPLE ARE ALWAYS FRIENDLY AND JOLLY, BECAUSE THEY CAN'T FIGHT OR RUN.

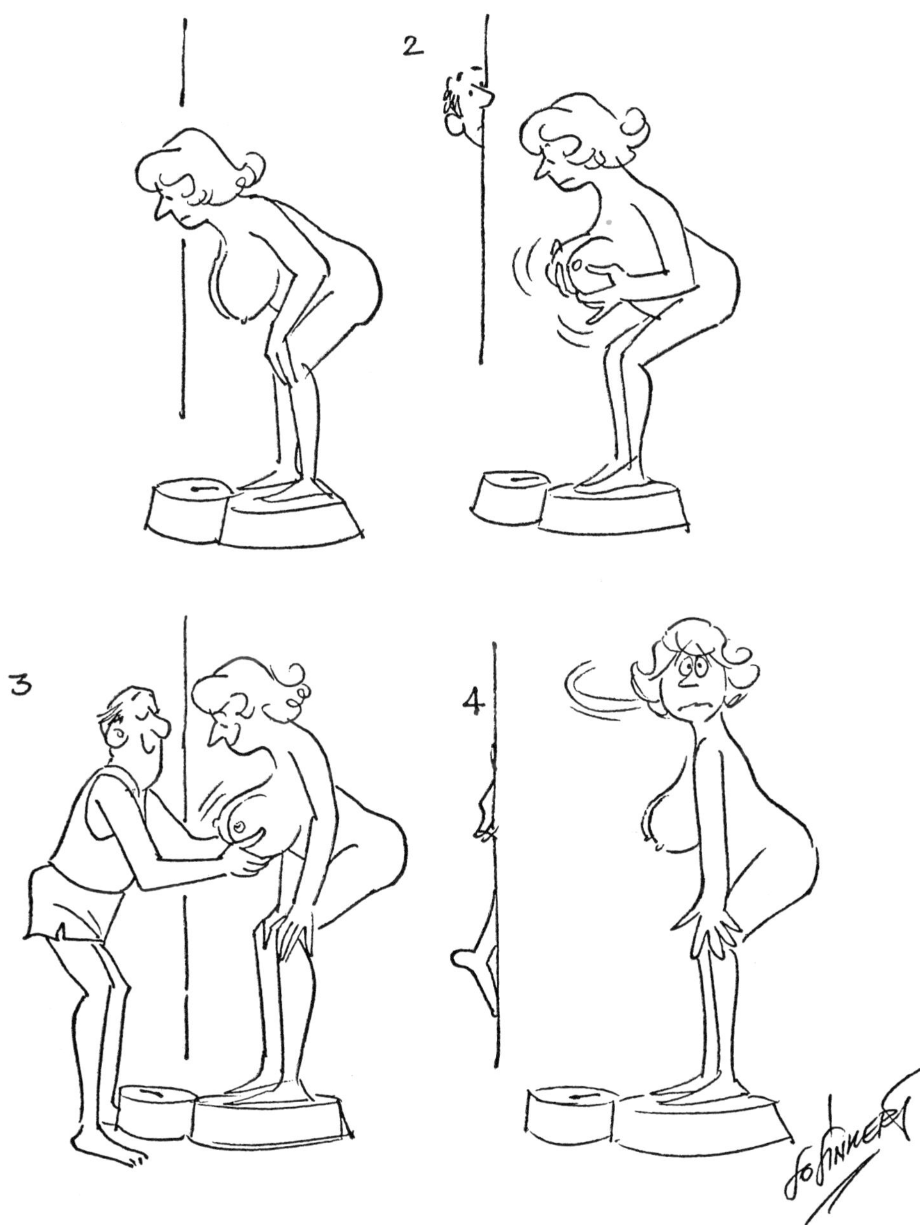
2
3
4

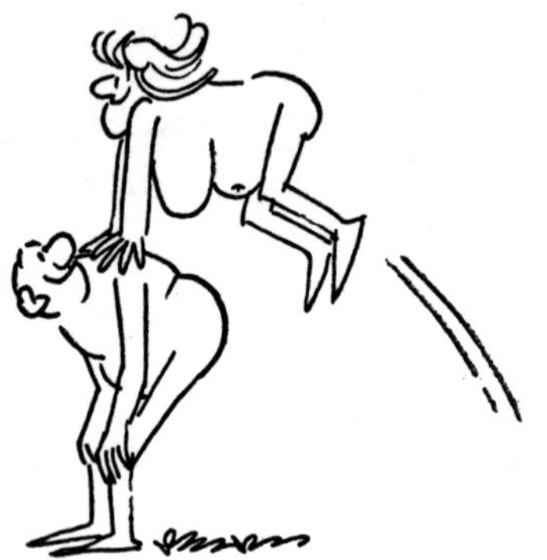

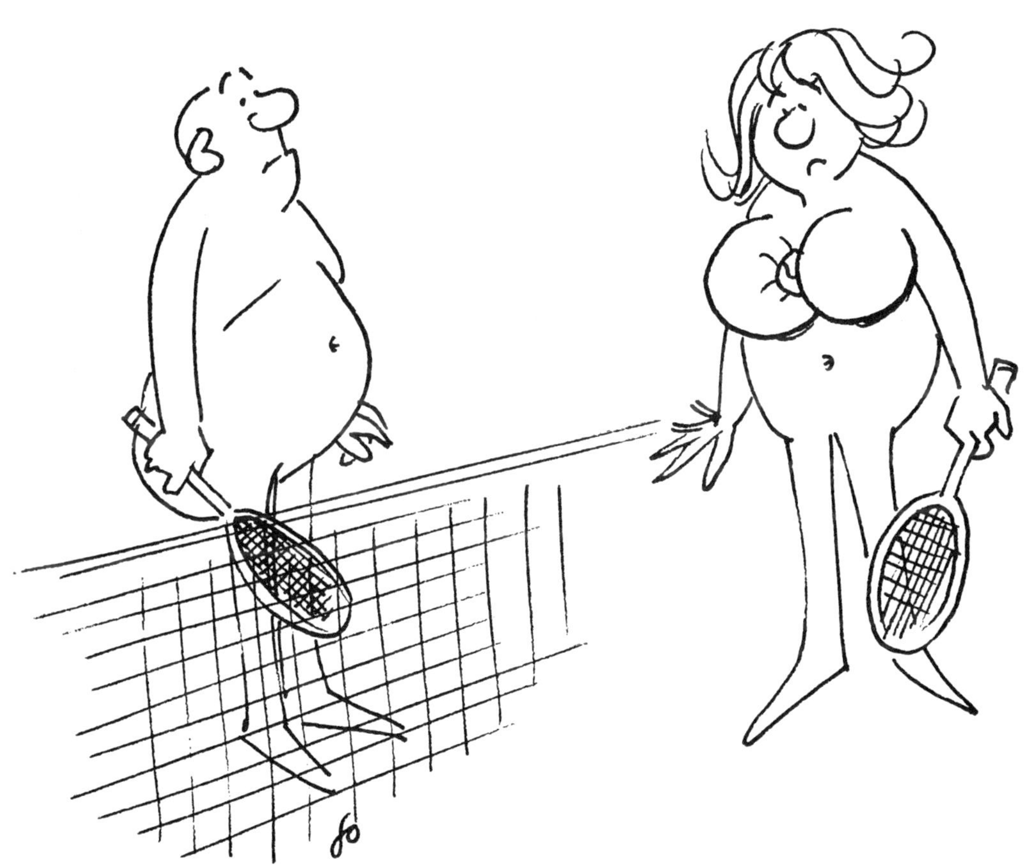

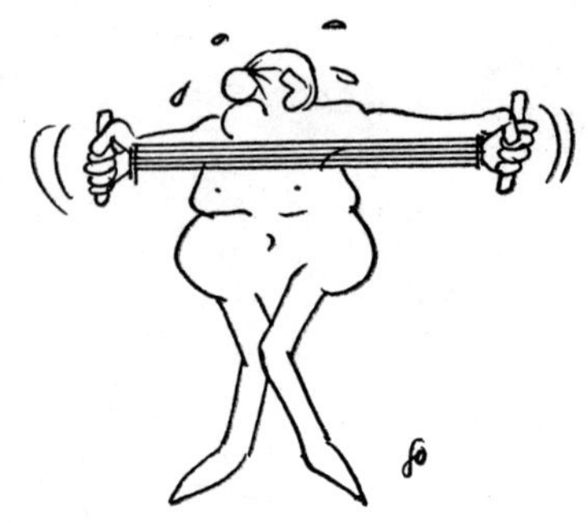

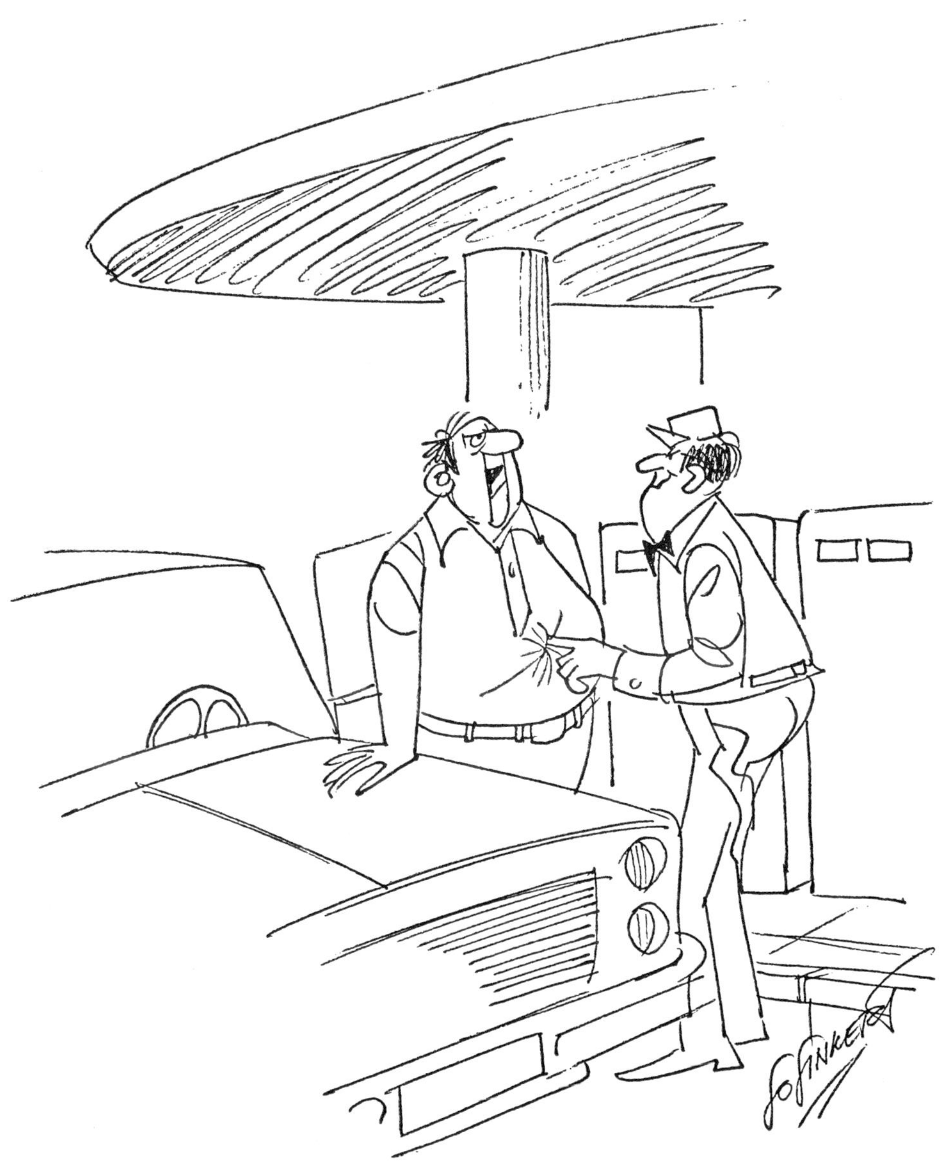

"THAT'S NOT WHAT I MEANT WHEN I ASKED YOU TO CHECK MY SPARE."

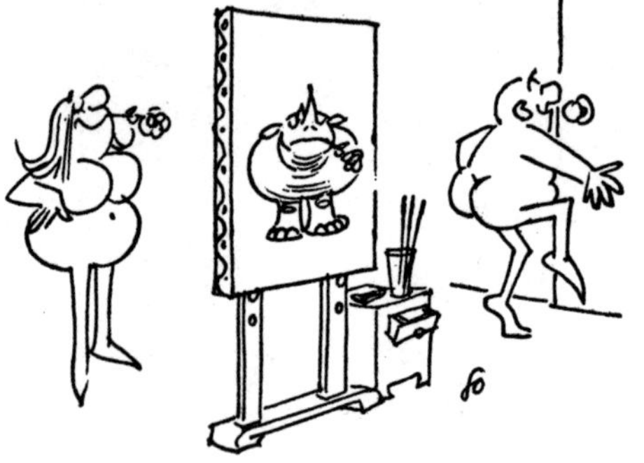

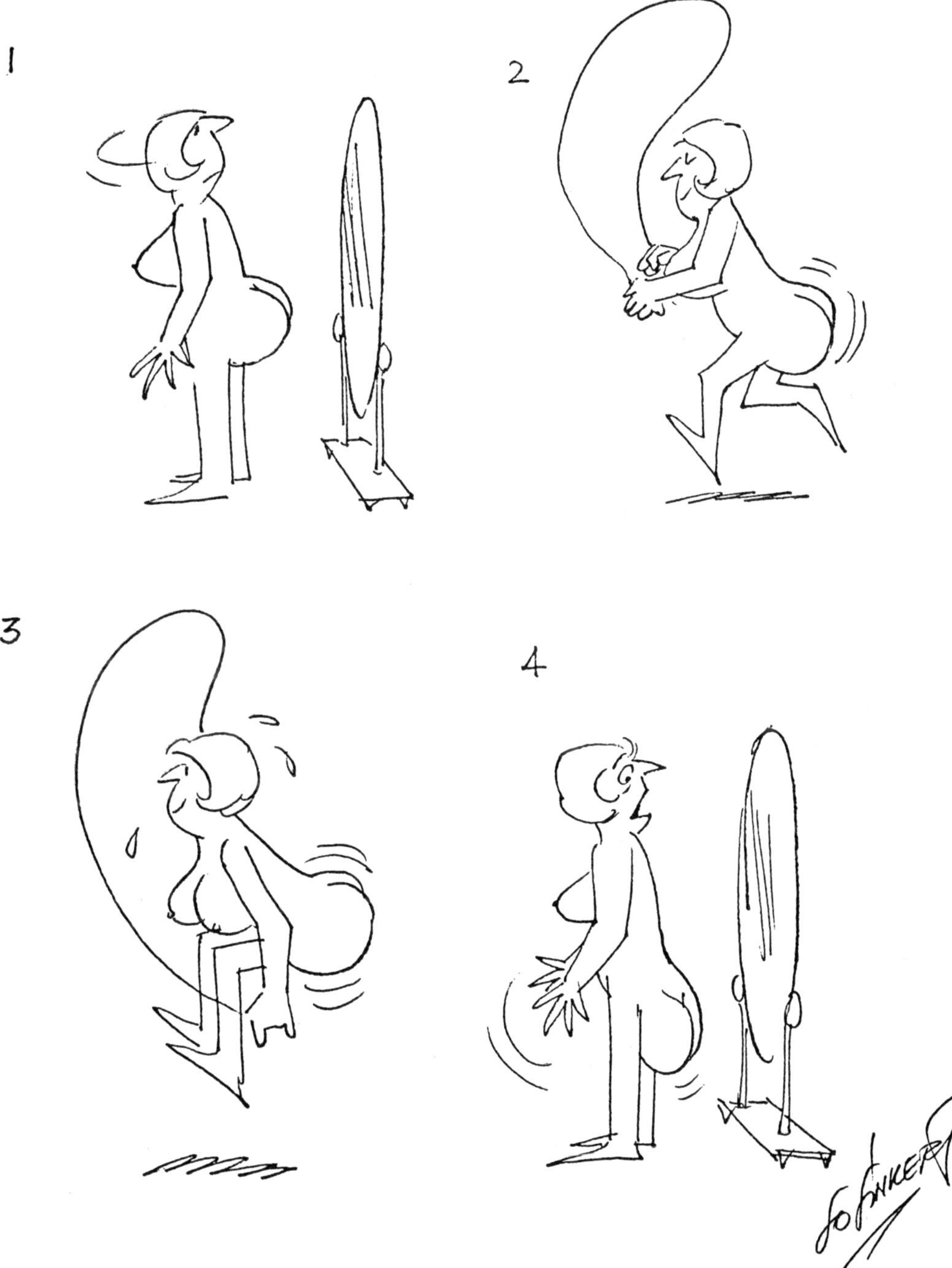
1
2
3
4

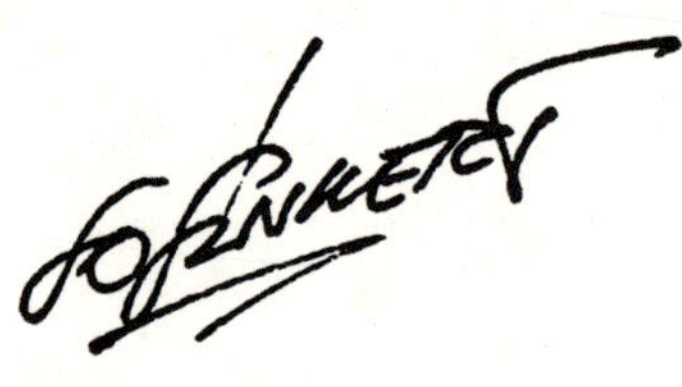

CARTOON SERIES

Golftoons

For Golftoons, Lo has selected his best golf cartoons, placing them under one cover. His hilarious talking golf ball is liberally sprinkled throughout the text. Lo's best barbs, however, are directed towards the frustrated duffer who suffers momentary lapses in etiquette. This is a book that every golfer will enjoy — on the 19th hole, in the locker room, or in the comfort of an easy chair by the fire.

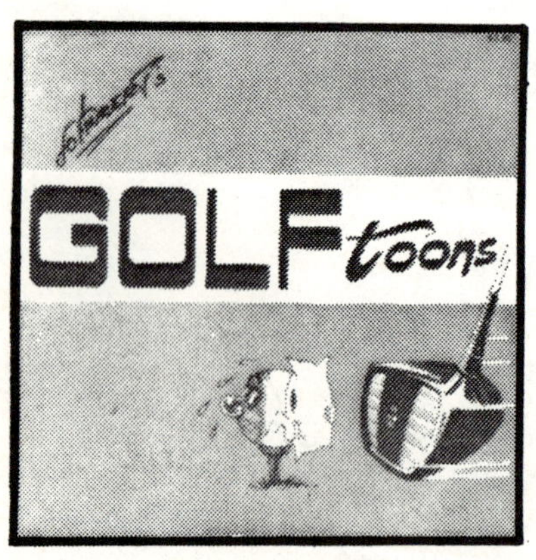

Hunters, Fishermen and Other Liars

Visual humor from "The World's Unluckiest Fisherman" guaranteed to keep you in stitches even if you have never hunted, fished or told "the truth.'

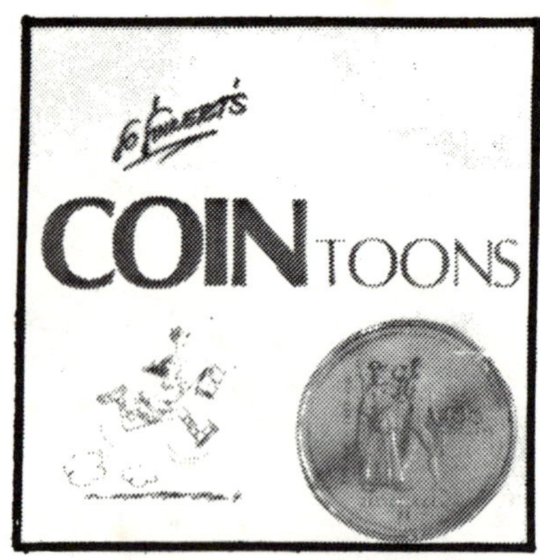

Cointoons

Cartoons with dollars, francs, kroners and pfennigs are no easy task, but Lo has come up with some first-class humor.

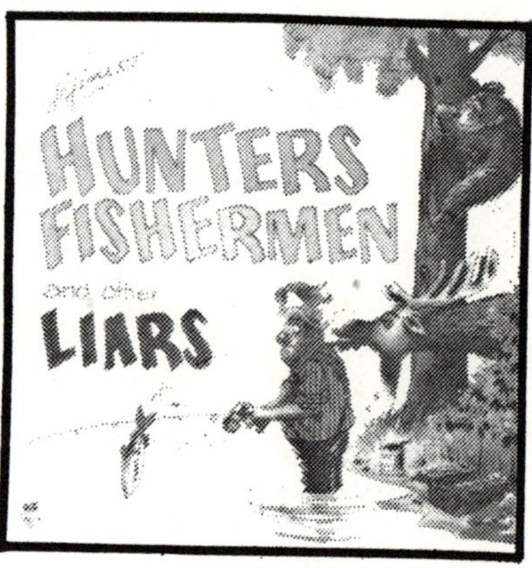

Also by Lo Linkert:
Stamptoons (German only)
Golftoons Calendar
Golftoons Posters

Look for these items in your bookstore or write to the publisher, **Plainsman Publications Ltd., 2133 Quebec St., Vancouver, B.C., Canada V5T 2Z9.**

In the United States:
The John Olson Company
294 West Oakland Avenue
Oakland, New Jersey 07436